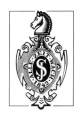

Sven-Erik Bergentz · David Bergqvist

Iatrogenic Vascular Injuries

With 52 Figures and 24 Tables

Springer-Verlag Berlin Heidelberg NewYork
London Paris Tokyo

Prof. Sven-Erik Bergentz
Ass. Prof. David Bergqvist
University of Lund, Dept. of Surgery,
Malmö General Hospital, S – 21401 Malmö

ISBN 3-540-50308-0 Springer-Verlag Berlin Heidelberg New York
ISBN 0-387-50308-0 Springer-Verlag New York Berlin Heidelberg

Library of Congress Cataloging-in-Publication Data
Bergentz, Sven-Erik.
Iatrogenic vascular injuries/Sven-Erik Bergentz, David Bergqvist.
Includes index.
ISBN 0-387-50308-0 (U.S.: alk. paper)
1. Blood-vessels – Wounds and injuries. 2. Therapeutics-Complications and sequelae. 3. Iatrogenic
diseases. I. Bergqvist, David, 1941. II. Title.
[DNLM: 1. Blood Vessels – injuries. 2. Iatrogenic Disease. WG 500 B4951] RD598.5.B47
1989 617'.413044 – dc 19 DNLM/DLC

Typesetting: Brühlsche Universitätsdruckerei, Giessen
Offsetprinting: Saladruck, Berlin. Bookbinding: Lüderitz & Bauer, Berlin
2121/3030-543210 – Printed on acid-free paper

Foreword

This small but information-packed book is the first to focus exclusively on iatrogenic vascular injuries. It is a timely first, for the scope and magnitude of this subject have reached almost epidemic proportions recently, as a result of exponential increases in the use of invasive diagnostic and therapeutic procedures by almost every medical and surgical speciality.

The data on vascular trauma from "civilian" experiences are becoming dominated by injuries of iatrogenic cause. Even were it not for medical-legal liability, the importance of prompt recognition and correct treatment of injuries that we ourselves cause is obvious, as is the need for preventive measures to be clearly identified and adopted. This book serves these needs well through a nicely balanced focus on prevention, on the one hand, with its comprehensive review of epidemiology and etiology, and on management, on the other, with its practical comments on diagnosis, treatment and outcome.

The organization of this book makes it very usable. After chapters on both arterial and venous catheterization injuries, there follows a thorough analysis of injuries associated with percutaneous transluminal angioplasty and other endovascular procedures. Then, after a chapter on noninvasive vascular injuries, there follows a series of chapters dealing with vascular injuries associated with the practice of specific specialties: radiation therapy, orthopedics, neurosurgery (especially lumbar disc surgery), gynecology, head and neck surgery, urology, adult general surgery, and pediatric surgery.

The authors are to be congratulated on building from the unique perspective which the Swedish system of reporting these iatrogenic injuries affords and, through a thorough literature review, creating for us a global view of this growing problem.

Denver, January 1989   Robert B. Rutherford

Contents

Preface

The amount of literature on vascular surgery is increasing dramatically, but so far no textbook has been published that deals exclusively with iatrogenic vascular injuries. Although some review articles have appeared, the problems concerning iatrogenic vascular trauma have not received appropriate attention in current textbooks on the vascular system. We therefore think it worthwhile to summarize present knowledge on this subject. Other important reasons for dealing with iatrogenic vascular trauma are their increasing frequency and the necessity of an optimal plan of action, particularly since the injury has been inflicted by us. Moreover, iatrogenic vascular injuries may occur at any time and without warning during various types of interventions and almost always require urgent handling. This means that any surgeon can be confronted by this problem.

In determining the limits of our presentation, we have excluded stenotic lesions occurring after kidney transplantation, vascular injuries inflicted by aortic balloon counterpulsation and by vascular surgery, and vascular damage induced by pharmacologic substances. Venous injuries will be considered in the various chapters, but deep vein thrombosis will be dealt with only occasionally.

One of us (Sven-Erik Bergentz) has served as an expert to the Swedish Board of Health and Welfare and its Responsibility Board for more than 15 years. Sweden has a rather unique law requiring all medical personnel to report mishaps occurring in hospitals, in which patients have been injured or endangered. As an expert adviser, he has had the opportunity to analyze a number of iatrogenic vascular injuries reported to these authorities. Some of them have been published (in Swedish) in *Läkartidningen* and in a monograph on litigation in surgery and orthopedics in cooperation with Professor Göran Bauer (1986)[1]. Since no report has been made in a foreign language before, we have used some of these cases to illustrate important points in this monograph.

Our secreteries Birgit Alm and Marie-Louise Strömberg are greatly acknowledged.

---

[1] Bauer G, Bergentz S-E (1985) När skyddsnätet brister. Lärdomar från sjukvårdens ansvarsnämnd. Studentlitteratur, Lund

Introduction

Adances in medicine have created a large number of invasive methods that are very helpful in diagnosis, monitoring, and treatment. A continuously increasing number of patients are being exposed to these techniques and are thereby at risk for iatrogenic vascular complications. These vascular complications vary in severity, but they unfortunately can be fatal or lead to limb loss and must frequently be handled on an urgent basis. Of 49 cases leading to litigation after vascular surgery, iatrogenic vascular emergencies occurred in 12 (Bergan 1987). In eight cases the cause was one of various types of arterial catheterization. Natali and Benhamou (1979) collected 125 cases of vasular injuries, excluding angiographic, during their 20 years of experience as experts with a French medical insurance company and as court witnesses. Nineteen of the injuries were iatrogenic (Table 1), and there were 32 cases of Volkman's syndrome in the upper extremity after fracture treatment; of these, 20 had circular plaster and eight had ischemia after lower-limb plaster treatment.

"Iatrogenic" comes from the Greek word for the art of healing – *iatreia*. Iatrogenic injury may be defined as any injury caused by a medical intervention or encounter. The problems posed by iatrogenic injuries are difficult to analyze and probably rather extensively underestimated because of the lack of an exact defi-

Table 1. Number and type of vascular injuries among 125 cases reported by Natali and Benhamou (1979)

Type of procedure	Number of vascular injuries	Number of injuries relevant to this discussion
Varicose vein surgery	12	6 arterial lesions (5 amputations) 1 arterial stripping (reconstruction) 1 venous laceration (death)
Arterial surgery	4	
General surgery	2	1 pseudoaneurysm after groin hernia
Orthopedic surgery	35	2 arm osteosynthesis (amputation) 1 femoral osteotomy, a. femoralis superficial (amputation) 1 meniscectomy, a. poplitea (chronic ischemia)
Arterial puncture	70	1 pseudoaneurysm, a. femoralis after blood sampling 4 i. a. infusion, a. femoralis in children 1 aortic puncture (rupture)
Laparoscopy	2	
	125	19

nition and the lack of systems for reporting and categorizing them. Medical intervention can refer either to drugs or to medical or surgical procedures. The indication for an encounter can be diagnosis, prophylaxis, or therapy. Stell et al. (1981), for example, defined iatrogenic illness as any illness resulting from a diagnostic procedure or from any form of therapy. They also included harmful occurrences that were not the natural consequences of the patient's disease.

Three main difficulties concerning iatrogenic diseases are the determination of prevalence and incidence, the cause-effect relationship, and the severity. In the total panorama of iatrogenic diseases and complications, vascular injuries are rare (Justiniani 1984; Lakshmanan et al. 1986; Trunet et al. 1982). This is also true of fatal cases. From a coroner's office in Dayton, Ohio, Murphy (1986) reported therapeutic misadventures in 44 of 9497 cases (0.46%). Of these, five were fatal hemorrhages because of vascular or visceral operative trauma, two were vascular or cardiac lacerations during diagnostic procedures, and one was a vascular laceration during some unspecified therapeutic procedure; thus, at the most there were eight cases of iatrogenic vascular injury (18%). Steel et al. (1981) analyzed iatrogenic illness in all new patients admitted to two floors (83 beds) of a university medical service during a 5-month period in 1979. A total of 815 patients were seen, 290 (36%) having a total of 497 iatrogenic illnesses. Of these 45 were seen after cardiac catheterization. However, a more detailed analyzis is not possible from the data in the publication. Fear of litigation may be responsible for underreporting. When potentially dangerous injuries are dealt with lege artis, leaving no sequelae, they tend to be forgotten and not reported in diagnostic registries. All retrospective data on frequencies must therefore be considered with caution.

There are many ways to classify iatrogenic injuries, each method having its advantages and drawbacks: anatomic localization, mechanism of injury, and consequence of injury. From the purely technical point of view, Adar et al. (1982) classified iatrogenic complications as resulting from:
1. Accident
2. Faulty technique or routine
3. Error in judgement or management
4. Failure to correctly identify anatomical structures, or failure to correctly interpret radiographs or laboratory findings
    The same authors also made a classification on the basis of the severity of the complication:
1. Severe – causing death, a life-threatening situation, major amputation, or severe disability
2. Moderate – causing mild permanent disability, complication requiring surgery or considerable prolongation of hospital stay
3. Mild – causing added discomfort and a short prolongation of hospital stay
    Except for numerous case reports and some review articles on special problems, iatrogenic vascular injuries have not received much attention. They nonetheless constitute a substantial part of vascular traumata in series with civilians suffering from vascular injuries. For instance, in the city of Malmö, Sweden, there has been a clear increase in such injuries during a 30-year period (Fig. 1). In Sweden, where vascular trauma due to interpersonal violence is still rare, the relative importance of iatrogenic injuries is great, but it must be emphasized that

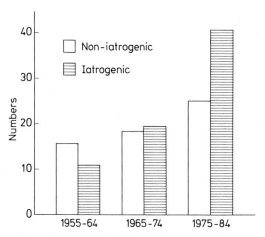

Fig. 1. Numbers of iatrogenic (▤) and noniatrogenic vascular injuries (☐) in three 10-year periods (1955–1984) at the Department of Surgery, Malmö General Hospital, Sweden. (From Acta Chir Scand 1987, 153: 417–422 with permission)

Table 2. Number and frequency of iatrogenic vascular injuries in reported series

Author	Year	Hospital, city	Period	No. of injuries	No. of iatrogenic injuries	Frequency (%)
Naely et al.	1961	Jackson	1955–1966	43	4	9
Owens	1963	Denver	1953–1962	70	20	29
Smith et al.	1963	Detroit	?	61	8	13
Thomford and Marable	1968	Columbus, Ohio	1953–1967	88	11	13
Moore et al.	1971	Galveston		250	25	10
Hardy et al.	1975	Jackson, Miss.	1957–1974	353	20	6
Kelly and Eisemann	1975	Denver	1971–1974	143	37	26
Shaker et al.[a]	1976	Baltimore	1965–1975	118	41	58
Whitehouse et al.[b]	1976	Ann Arbor	1965–1976	21	12	57
Kjellström and Risberg	1980	Gothenburg	1969–1978	82	14	17
Paaske et al.	1980	Copenhagen	1967–1978	42	0	0
Adar et al.	1982	Tel-Aviv	1978–1980	72	55	76
Thomas and Baird	1983	Bristol	1974–1980	63	6	9.5
Feliciano et al.	1984	Houston	1982	456	14	3
Leblanc et al.[b]	1985	Toronto	1966–1981	48	40	83
Sharma et al.	1985	New York	1968–1978	211	3	1.4
Lantsberg et al.	1986	Beer-Sheva	1973–1983	57	2	4
Bergqvist et al.	1987	Malmö	1955–1984	130	72	55

[a] Children under 15 years of age.
[b] Children under 18 years of age.

Table 3. Etiology of iatrogenic vascular injuries in some representative series

Reference	Total no.	Cardiac catheterization	Angio-graphy	Surgery[a]	Other
Buri (1971)	49	7	12	25	5
Hofmann et al. (1974)	17	1	6	7	3
Rich et al. (1974)	82	32	25	22	3
Rostan and Loup (1978)	24		12	12	2
Pietri et al. (1981)	44		27	27	1
Youkey et al. (1983)	119	35	40	34	10
Orcutt et al.[a] (1985)	22	9	6	4	3
Mills et al. (1986)	71	44	10	10	10
Bergqvist et al. (1987)	71	12	30	30	
	499	140	168	171	37

[a] Cardiovascular surgery excluded.

they constitute a worldwide problem of increasing importance. In Table 2 data are listed from a number of publications on vascular trauma; they show the great variations existing between different series. The studies on vascular injuries in children show a very high frequency of iatrogenicity (Leblanc et al. 1985; Shaker et al. 1976; Whitehouse et al. 1976). A high frequency is also seen in the only truly prospective study on vascular trauma (Adar et al. 1982).

Table 3 shows the etiologic panorama in some series which deal to a great extent with iatrogenic vascular injuries. As can be expected, angiography dominates, followed by an equal number of injuries caused by cardiac catheterization and surgery. In 1968, Vollmar published a series of iatrogenic vascular injuries, but he also included those occurring during vascular surgery, and in his publication it is not possible to distinguish these from the other types of injuries.

There are several factors of principal importance for the occurrence of iatrogenic vascular injuries; the main factors are related to the doctor or are found in the patient.

The Doctor

1. Insufficient knowledge – This is rather obvious but nonetheless important to consider. Safe surgery is very much a matter of proper knowledge of topographic anatomy. An example is the venous and arterial anatomy in the fossa ovalis, which now and then causes problems in varicose vein surgery. Another is the pelvic vascular anatomy in cases of extensive gynecologic surgery.
2. Failure to perform an anatomic dissection – It is important, when dissecting in the vicinity of vessels, not to protrude through the adventital layer; this can sometimes be difficult, especially when the tissue is scarred from previous surgery or has been irradiated.
3. Traumatic technique – An example of this is the blind application of clamps when groin bleeding occurs in varicose vein surgery.

4. Faulty technique – Examples are the performance of laparoscopy in an insufficiently insufflated abdominal cavity or puncture of the posterior wall of the femoral-iliac artery above the inguinal ligament at arterial catheterization.

The Patient

The first three points are rather obvious and will not be discussed further.
1. Inflammation
2. Tumor
3. Irradiation (which may also cause vessel injury in itself; see p.63)
4. Reoperation – The presence of scar tissue and sometimes distortion of normal vessel anatomy increase the risk of the occurrence of vascular trauma. Thus, reoperation in the hip region or for lumbar disk herniation is significantly more likely to induce vascular injury than are primary operations.
5. Anatomic variations – These are abundant, not all being of importance. Examples of variants which may cause trouble are aberrant hepatic and renal arteries. Another is Riolan's anastomosis, which is important to recognize during large bowel surgery. Today there are also an increasing number of patients who have previously been arterially reconstructed, some of them with extra-anatomic bypasses. These iatrogenic anatomic variations are important to consider when performing other surgical procedures within the field of former reconstruction. It would be desirable to contact vascular surgeons and to discuss with them how to minimize the risk of damaging the reconstruction.

It can be considered a truism that a physician's knowledge of iatrogenic injuries and of how to handle them must be optimal, as they are inflicted by us. They often place the patient in a very urgent situation and create a higher surgical risk, and the sequelae may be disastrous if primary treatment is inadequate.

It is important to remember that iatrogenic injuries may occur even in the best hands. We can never, even using modern and sophisticated medical techniques, hope to completely avoid iatrogenic vascular injuries. We therefore need knowledge of the various types of injuries that occur, and we need a proper plan for diagnosing and handling them. Through proper management of such injuries most of their harmful consequences can be eliminated.

References

Adar R, Bass A, Walden R (1982) Iatrogenic complications in surgery. Five years' experience in general and vascular surgery in a university hospital. Ann Surg 196:725–729
Bergan JJ (1987) Litigation after acute vascular emergencies. In: Bergan JJ, Yao JST (eds) Vascular surgical emergencies. Grune and Stratton, New York pp 43–54
Bergqvist D, Helfer M, Jensen N, Tägil M (1987) Trends in civilian vascular trauma during 30 years. Acta Chir Scand 153:417–422
Buri (1971) Iatrogene Schädigung von Blutgefäßen. Helv Chir Acta 38:151–155
Feliciano D, Bitondo CG, Mattox KL et al. (1984) Civilian trauma in the 1980s. A 1-year experience with 456 vascular and cardiac injuries. Ann Surg 199:717–724
Hardy JD, Raju S, Neely WA, Berry DW (1975) Aortic and other arterial injuries. Ann Surg 181:640–653

Hofmann K-T, Simonis G, Männl HFK, Kock B (1974) Iatrogene Verletzungen der großen Gefäße und am Herzen. Munch Med Wochenschr 116:975–982

Justiniani FR (1974) Iatrogenic disease: an overview. MT Sinai J Med (NY) 51:210–214

Kelly GL, Eiseman B (1975) Civilian vascular injuries. J Trauma 15:507–514

Kjellström T, Risberg B (1980) Vascular trauma. Review of 10 years' experience. Acta Chir Scand 146:261–265

Lakshmanan M, Hershey C, Breslau D (1986) Hospital admissions caused by iatrogenic disease. Arch Intern Med 146:1931–1934

Lantsberg L, Golcman L, Khodadadi Z et al. (1986) Arterial injuries in the civilian and military population. Clin Eur J Clin Exp Med Surg 3:1–3

Leblanc J, Wood A, O'Shea M, Williams W, Trusler G, Rowe R (1985) Peripheral arterial trauma in children. A fifteen-year review. J Cardiovasc Surg 28:325–331

Mills JL, Wiedeman JE, Robinson JG, Hallett JW (1986) Minimizing mortality and morbidity from iatrogenic arterial injuries: the need for early recognition and prompt repair. J Vasc Surg 4:22–27

Moore CG, Wolma FJ, Brown RW, Derrick JR (1971) Vascular trauma: a review of 250 cases. Am J Surg 122:576

Murphy GK (1986) Therapeutic misadventure. An 11-year study from a metropolitan coroner's office. Am J Forensic Med Pathol 7:115–119

Naely W, Hardy J, Artz C (1961) Arterial injuries in civilian practice: a current reappraisal with analysis of forty-three cases. J Trauma 1:424–439

Natali J, Benhamou AC (1979) Iatrogenic vascular injuries. A review of 125 cases (excluding angiographic injuries). J Cardiovasc Surg (Torino) 20:169–176

Orcutt MB, Levine BA, Gaskill HV, Sirinek KR (1985) Iatrogenic vascular injury. A reducible problem. Arch Surg 120:384–385

Owens JC (1963) The management of arterial trauma. Surg Clin North Am 43:371–385

Paaske WP, Lorentzen JE, Buchardt-Hansen HJ (1980) Peripheral arterial injuries. Acta Chir Scand [Suppl] 502:176–180

Pietri P, Alagni G, Settembrini PG, Gabrielli F (1981) Iatrogenic vascular lesions. Int Surg 66:213–216

Rich NM, Hobson RW, Fedde CW (1974) Vascular trauma secondary to diagnostic and therapeutic procedures. Am J Surg 128:715–721

Rostan O, Loup P (1978) Lésions vasculaires iatrogènes. Rev Med Suisse Romande 98:321–327

Shaker IJ, White JJ, Signer RD, Golladay ES, Haller JA (1976) Special problems of vascular injuries in children. J Trauma 16:863–867

Sharma PV, Babu SC, Shah PM, Clauss RH (1985) Changing patterns in civilian arterial injuries. J Cardiovasc Surg 26:7–11

Smith RF, Szilagyi DE, Pfeifer JR (1963) Arterial trauma. Arch Surg 86:153–163

Steel K, Gertman PM, Crescenzi C, Anderson (1981) Iatrogenic illness on a general medical service at a university hospital. N Engl J Med 304:638–642

Thomas WEG, Baird RN (1983) Arterial injuries in two Bristol hospitals from 1974 to 1980. Injury 15:30–34

Thomford NR, Marable SA (1968) Arterial trauma. A review of 88 acute injuries. Chicago State Med J 64:1143–1148

Trunet P, Le Gall JR, Lhoste F, Rapin M (1982) Admissions to intensive care units for iatrogenic diseases. Leg Med 73–84

Vollmar J (1968) Iatrogene Gefäßverletzungen in der Chirurgie. Langenbecks Arch Klin Chir 322:335–339

Whitehouse W, Coran A, Stanley J, Kuhns L, Weintraub W, Fry W (1976) Pediatric vascular trauma. Manifestations, management, and sequelae of extremity arterial injury in patients undergoing surgical treatment. Arch Surg 111:1269–1275

Youkey JR, Clagett GP, Rich NM et al. (1983) Vascular trauma secondary to diagnostic and therapeutic procedures: 1974 through 1982. Am J Surg 146:788–791

Injuries Caused by Diagnostic Arterial Catheterization or Puncture

Types of Injury

Arterial catheterization or puncture may cause (a) major bleeding, indicated by hematoma or shock, (b) occlusion or stenosis due to thromboembolism or intimal injury, (c) arteriovenous fistula, or (d) pseudoaneurysm, true aneurysm, or arterial wall dissection, and (e) may leave a foreign body in the arterial system, such as fragments of guide wires or fractured tips of catheters. In addition, it has been suggested that toxic effects of angiographic contrast media might cause occlusion of stenotic arteries, unrelated to the effect of the catheter (van Andel 1980). Toxic injury caused by contrast media to parenchymatous organs (kidneys, liver, brain, spinal cord, etc.) will not be discussed.

Causes of Injury

Hemorrhage is a regular phenomenon after arterial puncture, but it is usually local and minor. Major hemorrhage may be caused by perforation of the back wall of the artery, which is difficult to compress, particularly in the retroperitoneal area. In these cases, the blood loss may be great enough to cause hypovolemic shock, due to the very loose tissue with absence of counterpressure and lack of initial local symptoms.

Factors contributing to excessive blood loss are multiple punctures, particularly if both the front and back wall of the artery are perforated, a large catheter diameter, and anticoagulation therapy (Antonovic et al. 1976; Illescas et al. 1986; McEnany and Austen 1977, Neviaser et al. 1976). Massive hemorrhage may also occur from inadvertent arterial lesion during venous catheterization. One example is attempted insertion of a balloon-tipped pulmonary artery catheter via the internal jugular vein, perforating the carotid arteries (Civetta et al. 1972).

Hemorrhage may also be due to perforation of the aorta or any peripheral artery by the tip of the catheter (Imoto et al. 1985). The risk is particularly high in infants, who have fragile arteries (Aguilar et al. 1966).

Thromboemboli may have one of two causes: The *first* is formation of platelet aggregates and fibrin on the surface of the catheter and in the holes on the catheter tip (Schlossman 1973; Wilner et al. 1978; Fig. 1). When the catheter is pulled out, the fibrin material is washed off on the inner side of the vessel, forming a small or a large thrombotic plug (Jacobsson et al. 1969 a, b). This thrombotic material may occasionally occlude the artery, but usually it forms a wall-adherent, nonocclusive thrombus (Fig. 2). In the former case the thrombus may prop-

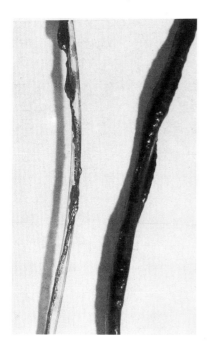

Fig. 1. Platelet aggregation and fibrin on the surface of angiography catheters

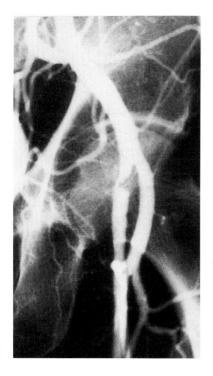

Fig. 2. Small, nonocclusive thrombus at the puncture site after catheter angiography

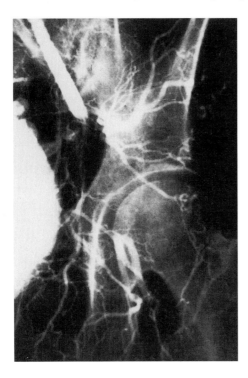

Fig. 3. Occlusive thrombus at the puncture site after catheter angiography

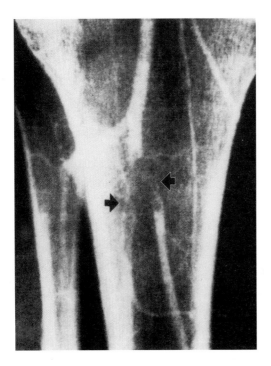

Fig. 4. Distal embolization (*arrows*) to the tibiofibular trunk after angiography with femoral artery puncture

agate proximally or distally (Fig. 3); in the latter, the thrombotic material may embolize distally (Fig. 4). By "pull-out arteriography", injection of contrast medium at the time the catheter is withdrawn, Antonovic et al. (1976) found that heparinization significantly decreased the amount of thrombotic material collected on the catheter. Jacobsson et al. (1969a) and Schlossman (1973) demonstrated experimentally that the amount of thrombotic material depends on the type of catheter material but also that it increases with increasing length and width of the catheter as well as with the duration of catheterization.

Thrombotic material formed in the holes on the tip of the catheter may embolize if the catheter is flushed or when contrast medium is injected. This embolization may occlude various peripheral arteries or arterial branches when selective angiography is performed (Coddon and Krieger 1958; McAfee and Willson 1956; Harrington et al. 1968; Lang 1963; Lonni et al. 1969).

The *second* mechanism by which thromboembolic complication may occur is intimal rupture or dissection, or dislodgement of thrombotic or atherosclerotic material, either at the place of catheter insertion or by injury to the arterial wall caused by the tip of the catheter, particularly in selective catheterization (Andersen 1969; Baum and Eufrate 1962; Delin et al. 1979; Gill et al. 1972; Head and Robboy 1972; McDowell and Thompson 1959; Takolander et al. 1985; Fig. 5). Intimal dissection may cause an *immediate* occlusion, but it may also cause the progressive formation of a thrombus on the damaged intima, resulting in an occlusion or embolization after several hours or even days (Fogarty and Krippaehne 1965). Sometimes the intimal injury is severe but no occlusion occurs and the clinical course is uneventful (Fig. 6).

Arteriovenous fistulae are caused by simultaneous perforation of an artery and a vein. The formation of such a fistula was well known at the time when venesection was a common therapeutic procedure, the first case having been described by Hunter (Callander 1920). In modern times, such fistulae have been described in the groin between the femoral artery and vein (Rossi et al. 1974), in the cubital fossa between the brachial artery and the cubital vein (Lalljee 1970), on the wrist between the radial artery and the adjacent vein (Ontell and Gauderer 1985), on the neck between the vertebral artery and the vein plexus surrounding this artery (Bergquist 1971; Bergström and Lodin 1966; Lester 1966), and after splenoportography between the splenic artery and vein (Chait and Margulies 1966). (Arteriovenous fistulae after kidney biopsies, after various surgical procedures, and after venous catheterization are described also.)

Pseudoaneurysms are found around the hole in the artery, particularly if the hole is relatively large. They are usually formed at the place of catheter insertion (Wagner 1963) but may also form around a hole made by the tip of the catheter in a peripheral vascular branch (Imoto et al. 1985). Pseudoaneurysms are usually small, having the size of a golf ball or a mandarin orange (Fig. 7). Pseudoaneurysms are particularly prone to form if there has been excessive bleeding, and especially when patients on anticoagulants or antiplatelet drugs are catheterized (Bergentz et al. 1966; Eriksson and Jorulf 1970; Perl et al. 1973).

True aneurysms are rarely caused by arterial catheterization. Such aneurysms have been described as a late sequela following subintimal injection of contrast medium (Boblitt et al. 1959; Chiavacci et al. 1976; Jonsson et al. 1977) and after

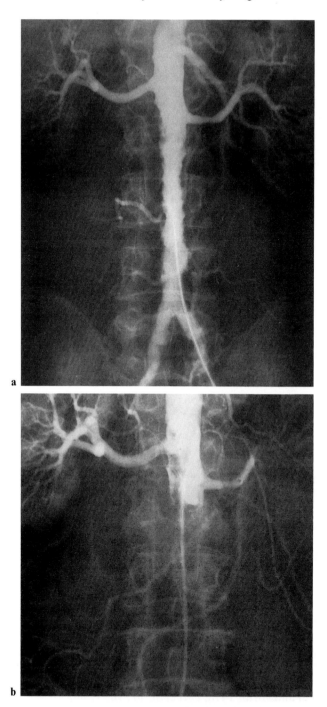

Fig. 5a, b. Aortography performed with Seldinger technique. **a** Severe aortic atherosclerosis is seen. **b** Subintimal dissection of the catheter has caused total occlusive thrombosis of the aorta distal to the renal arteries

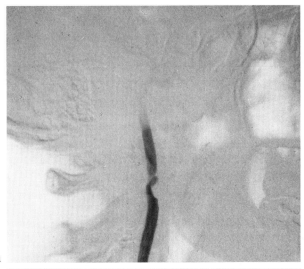

a

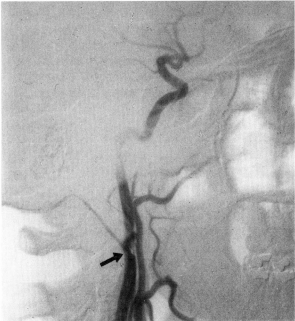

b

Fig. 6a, b. Intimal injury (*arrow*) in the internal carotid artery at selective angiography. There were no clinical manifestations related to this damage

multiple punctures of the radial artery for blood sampling (Mathieu et al. 1973). Infected aneurysms (so-called mycotic aneurysms) may occur following perforation of the intima with an infected tip of the catheter (Baker et al. 1979).

Dissection of the arterial wall with formation of a dissecting aneurysm occurs mainly after translumbar puncture or catheterization of the aorta, particularly if

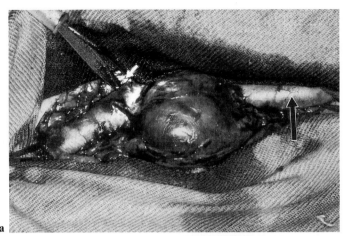

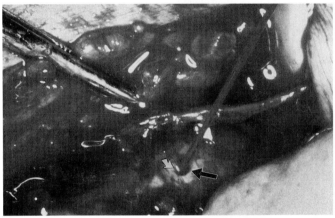

Fig. 7. a Pseudoaneurysm in the superficial femoral artery (*black arrow*) just distal to the deep femoral artery (*white arrow*). **b** *Arrows* point towards a small hole in the superficial femoral artery with a blood jet. Such a hole can mostly be closed with a simple suture

large volumes of contrast medium happen to be injected intramurally (Beall et al. 1964; Coran and Tyler 1968; Crawford et al. 1957; Gillanders 1963; Gudbjerg and Christensen 1961; Kocandrle et al. 1970). Intestinal circulation may be damaged by intramural contrast medium injection in translumbar angiography (Baum and Eufrate 1962; Guilfoil 1963; McDowell and Thomspon 1959; Puylaert 1965). The intima of peripheral arteries, such as the renal or the intestinal arteries, may be damaged by the tip of the catheter during selective catheterization (Andersen 1969; Bergentz et al. 1973; Engberg et al. 1974).

Fragmentation of the tip of the catheter or of the guide wire may occur during arterial catheterization. Parts of the catheter material may be lost and embolize (Blair et al. 1970; Bablitt et al. 1959).

Arterial damage from toxic effects of the contrast medium has been claimed to cause occlusions of stenotic areas of the arteries, but no definite proof has been given (van Andel 1980). It is not unlikely, however, that such lesions may occur, similar to the way in which thrombophlebitis is caused by phlebography. The modern, noniodinized contrast media should minimize this risk (Almén et al. 1977).

Incidence

Major complications have been defined as "complications threatening the life, limb, or visceral integrity of the patient, or requiring subsequent surgical intervention for diagnosis or treatment, or significantly prolonging the hospital stay of the patient" (Reiss et al. 1972). *Minor complications* have been described as "asymptomatic complication[s] of arteriography detected radiographically or a clinically insignificant transient symptom or sign, not endangering the patient or requiring further evaluation" (Reiss et al. 1972). A pragmatic way of defining major complications is to include complications requiring surgical intervention, plus fatal complications.

Since the frequency of complications is relatively low, it has been necessary to pool data from different articles or to survey data from different hospitals in order to properly evaluate the risks. Using such a technique in 1963, Lang surveyed 11 402 procedures of retrograde percutaneous *transfemoral* arteriography (Seldinger procedure), collecting data by sending out questionnaires to 300 hospital radiologists (Lang 1963). There were 81 (0.7%) major complications (requiring surgical intervention), including thrombosis, six of which resulted in loss of a limb. There were five cases of guide wire or catheter breakage and seven cases of major hematoma. Massive retroperitoneal hemorrhage from perforation of a pelvic artery occurred in three cases.

These figures were compared with data from another survey by Lang of 3240 patients undergoing *translumbar* aortography, which resulted in only 11 major complications, (0.3%), including four cases of retroperitoneal hemorrhage and two cases of bowel necrosis due to mesenteric thrombosis. The mortality was higher in the translumbar group, however, (0.28% versus 0.06%). In an early study from 1957, MacAfee (MacAfee 1957) reported results of a survey of 13 207 translumbar aortographies resulting in 98 major complications, such as neurological disturbances and bleeding complications (0.74%), and 37 deaths (0.28%).

In a more recent survey from 1981 Hessel and co-workers (Hessel et al. 1981) reported on complications of 118 591 angiographic examinations from a large number of hospitals, comparing *transfemoral, translumbar, and transaxillary* approaches. The overall complication rates were 1.73% for the transfemoral group, 2.89% for the translumbar group, and 3.29% for the transaxillary group. Thirty deaths were reported, with the highest incidence in the transaxillary group and the lowest in the transfemoral. In the transaxillary group there were also more neurological complications, including seizures and hemiplegia, but also more cases of hemorrhage, arterial obstruction, and pseudoaneurysm. In the translumbar group there were more cases of bleeding and of extraluminal contrast injection. The incidence of puncture-site thrombosis was 0.14% in the transfemoral group as compared with 0.6% in the transaxillary group and 0% in the translumbar group. Emboli occurred in 0.10% of the transfemoral group, 0.07%

of the transaxillary group, and 0% of the translumbar group. An interesting finding in the study of Hessel et al. is the fact that the complication rate was more than four times higher (2.7% versus 0.6%) in hospitals doing less than 200 than in those doing more than 800 angiographies. This difference was particularly marked in the nonteaching hospitals (2.9% versus 0.3%) but was negligible in the teaching hospitals (1.3% versus 0.8%).

Several other studies have reported figures similar to those given by Hessel et al. The translumbar technique using a needle or a catheter is often reported to cause relatively few but serious complications, such as bowel necrosis, aortic dissection (which may also cause intestinal gangrene), or major bleeding. Thromboembolic complications are rare, however, and definitely fewer than when the Seldinger technique is used.

There has been an obvious tendency during the past 10–15 years for fewer complications to occur in all types of arterial punctures and catheterizations. This is suggested by the reports just mentioned, but also by a series of prospective studies. In a survey reviewing 1000 consecutive cases of percutaneous *transfemoral* catheter angiographies, Halpern reported five (0.5%) cases of thrombotic occlusions, one (0.1%) case of pseudoaneurysm, two (0.2%) cases of fractured guide wire tips, and 17 (1.7%) of hematoma and bleeding problems (Halpern 1964). In a study of 9200 patients undergoing transfemoral catheter angiography, Eriksson and Jorulf (1970) reported 20 (0.22%) cases of thrombosis, ten pseudoaneurysms (0.11%), one broken guide wire (0.01%), and seven (0.07%) cases of bleeding complications. In a study of 1217 angiographies in which the Seldinger technique was used, Sigstedt and Lunderquist (1978) reported 0.14% complications at the puncture site requiring surgery. Our own experience confirms this tendency of a decreasing incidence of complications.

The *translumbar* technique, although used less frequently today, has also been characterized by a decreased incidence of complications. Szilagyi et al. (1977) reviewed their series of 14550 translumbar aortographies and reported an overall complication rate of 0.05% (seven cases) and two deaths (0.014%). These figures compare very favourably with those just quoted from McAffe's study from 1957.

The site of catheterization is of decisive importance for the incidence and type of complication. Several reports have confirmed the high frequency of complications following catheterization of the *axillary artery*. Staal et al. (1966) reported on 21 consecutive cases of arterial catheterization by the transaxillary approach. Five patients had slight disturbances from the brachial plexus, characterized as paresthesia and weakness, for some months. Two other patients had severe and irreversible lesions. Molnar and Paul (1972) presented 1762 consecutive cases with a complication rate of 2.1%. These included nine cases of local thrombosis, 11 cases of axillary hematoma with motor deficit, and three cases of pseudoaneurysm, one with a motor deficit. They concluded that puncture of the axillary artery is an attractive alternative percutaneous route whenever femoral introduction of the catheter is not feasible or is unsuccessful. Brachial plexus paralysis could be eliminated in most instances by a meticulus technique and by avoiding delay in surgical exploration once paresis has developed. Dudrik et al. (1967) reported two cases of plexus damage following 305 axillary arteriographies, also stressing the importance of immediate exploration to minimize neurologic deficit.

Field et al. (1987) reported a series of 102 patients in whom the arterial tree had been successfully visualized by transaxillary angiography. Two patients (1.9%) required embolectomy, and three (2.9%) showed transient neurologic deficit consistent with brachial plexus injury.

Catheterization of the *brachial artery* has been used as an alternative to axillary artery catheterization to avoid the risk of damage of the brachial plexus (Hall 1971; McCollum and Mavor 1986). Such catheterization, like catheterization of other peripheral arteries, can be done either by an open *cut-down technique* with open arteriotomy or by *percutaneous catheterization*. There seems to be a tendency to use the percutaneous technique more often in recent years. Several authors claim that catheter angiography is safer than open arteriotomy (Rubenson et al. 1979). No prospective comparative studies have been reported, however.

As early as 1957, Abrahams reported a case of gangrene affecting four fingers following brachial artery catheterization, and many radiologists recommend that this artery be avoided as a site for puncture. It is obvious that the number of thrombotic occlusions following brachial artery catheterization is higher than generally expected. Due to the excellent collateral circulation, however, occlusions often cause few or no symptoms. In the series of Feild et al. (1962) of 1202 brachial angiograms in which the percutaneous technique was used, there was no case of ischemia leading to amputation, but altogether the complication rate was 7.91%, 0.60% being classified as severe. Hall (1971) reported one case of below-elbow and one of above-elbow amputation following brachial artery catheterization, but the size of his total series is not clear. McCollum and Mavor (1986) reported 106 occlusions following 12 158 (0.9%) cardiac catheterizations of the brachial artery using open arteriotomy. Forty-two of these were discovered and reexplored by the cardiologists at the time of catheterization. Using the same technique, Campion et al. (1971) noticed pulse reduction in 42 of 342 arteriotomies. In 24 the arteriotomy was reopened with removal of a clot. In a prospective study, Barnes et al. (1978), using a Doppler ultrasound velocity detector, found occlusion of the brachial artery in 17% of patients, but two-thirds of these had no symptoms of ischemia.

Hammacher et al. (1988) did a careful prospective study of 502 patients before and after brachial arterial cardiac catheterization. Examination, palpation of pulse, Doppler waveform analysis, segmental blood pressure, and (if wrist blood pressure index was under 0.7) selective angiography were used as diagnostic methods. Twenty-nine patients (5.7%) had complaints of pain, pallor, or hypo- or paraesthesia and 39 (7.8%; not necessarily the same as those with symptoms) had a wrist index of under 0.7. Of these, 33 underwent angiography, 22 having occlusions and 11 stenoses. Significant risk factors found included previous catheterization and acquired heart disease. A wrist pressure index of 0.55 or less after exercise had the highest specificity and sensitivity in predicting arm claudication during follow-up.

It seems obvious that the risk for brachial artery occlusion, whatever technique is used, is relatively high in brachial artery catheterization (Bergentz 1988). This is probably due to the fact that the artery is narrow and that the upper limb arteries are more liable to spasm than those of the lower limb (Lindbom 1957;

Wickbom and Bartley 1957). The exact incidence of brachial artery occlusion is unknown, since many patients remain asymptomatic. Gangrene of the fingers is rare, and is probably most often due to peripheral embolic occlusions.

In operating rooms and intensive care units *radial artery cannulation* is often used to permit repeated arterial blood sampling and pressure recording. The cannulation can be performed either percutaneously or via an open arteriotomy. The catheter is often allowed to remain in place for several days, in constrast to most other peripheral artery catheters. In a prospective study of 100 such patients, with the catheter in place for a mean of 4 days, Cederholm et al. (1986) noted that not less than 33% had a thrombosis in the radial artery, as seen from disappearance of the radial pulse. In none of these patients were there any clinical symptoms of persisting finger ischemica. In the majority of the patients the radial artery thrombosis disappeared after removal of the catheter. Other authors, however, have reported persistent finger or hand ischemia and even gangrene after radial artery cannulation, requiring amputation of the hand or lower forearm, but the incidence is obviously variable (Downs et al. 1973; Falor et al. 1976; Miyasaka et al. 1976; Samaan 1971; Slogoff et al. 1983). Soderstrom et al. (1982) reported serious complications such as pseudoaneurysm, distal ischemia, or sepsis in 2.5% of their patients who had the catheter inserted for about 4 days. (In their series, transfemoral cannulation resulted in the same incidence of complications, but the catheters could be used for a longer time, or about 7 days). Samaan (1971) reported three cases of finger gangrene after 800 radial artery cannulations. It is recommended that Allen's test be carried out before the decision is made to catheterize this artery, thereby confirming that both the ulnar and radial artery are patent (Allen 1929; Brodsky 1975). According to Slogoff et al. (1983), however, the risk of permanent ischemia is very low, even if Allen's test shows occlusion of the ulnar or radial artery. On the other hand, normal results on the Allen's test do not exlude the possibility of permanent damage (Wilkins 1985). Risk factors for radial artery occlusion are female sex, low cardiac output, use of vasoconstrictor drugs, and preexisting peripheral arterial disease (Wilkins 1985).

The incidence of complications following *carotid artery puncture* for angiography has been difficult to establish, the reason being that the patients often have a serious cerebral or cerebrovascular disease, such as tumor, aneurysm, or hemorrhage (Amundsen et al. 1963; Coddon and Krieger 1958; Lindner et al. 1962; Perret and Nishioka 1966). The incidence of stroke was high in earlier publications, but probably this was most often due to the toxic effects of contrast medium (Coddon and Krieger 1958). Stroke due to carotid artery thrombosis, dissection, or embolization does occur (Lang 1966; Mani et al. 1978; Perret and Nishioka 1966). This is also true for ocular lesions from microemboli or from the contrast material (Falls et al. 1951; Haney and Preston 1962). Stroke has also been reported in six cases of accidental carotid artery puncture during internal jugular vein cannulation (Anagnous 1982; Civetta et al. 1972).

In carotid artery punctures, the *vertebral artery* is occasionally punctured accidentally. Vertebral artery puncture is also an established technique for vertebral angiography, but it is now rarely used. In the vertebral canal the vertebral artery is surrounded by a vein plexus (Batson's plexus; Fig. 8). At least 29 arteriovenous fistulae have been reported following vertebral artery catheterization (Bergentz

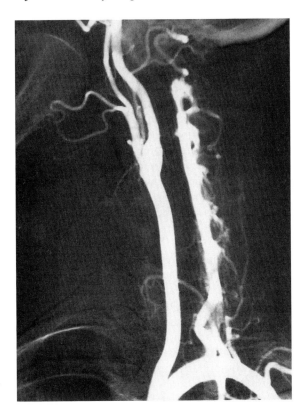

Fig. 8. A fistula between the vertebral artery and Batson's plexus after accidental vertebral artery puncture during carotid angiography

et al. 1966; Bergquist 1971; Björck 1966; Newton and Darroch 1966). Lester and Klee (1965) found two fistulae following 337 vertebral artery punctures, 34 of which occurred accidentally during carotid punctures.

Several cases of *renal artery* occlusion have been reported, particularly after selective catheterization of the renal artery. This may cause renal ischemia with impaired function of the kidney or renovascular hypertension (Bergentz et al. 1973; Engbert et al. 1974; Reiss et al. 1972). *Mesenteric* and *coeliac* artery occlusions have been described following selective catheterization of these arteries (Rutherford and Pearce 1987). Myocardial infarct from *coronary artery occlusion* has been found to occur following coronary angiography and heart catheterization (Moore et al. 1970; Takaro et al. 1972).

The incidence of more rare complications and the incidence of complications following more rarely used procedures are difficult to establish. In many situations there are only anecdotal reports.

Angiography in patients with *arterial grafts* is a special problem of increasing importance. Available data suggest that catheterization can be done through the graft wall without increased risk (Eisenberg et al. 1976).

Symptoms

Major hemorrhage may cause two different kinds of symptoms: local or general. The most common *local symptom* of hemorrhage is seen at the place of catheter insertion as an expanding, painful hematoma. In the axillary artery such a hematoma may cause brachial plexus compression with paresthesia, paresis, or paralysis of the arm, and in the carotid area, compression of the trachea and edema of the larynx (Feild and DeSaussure 1965). Major bleeding may cause *general symptoms* of hypovolemic shock. Such bleeding may come not from the place of catheter insertion, but from a perforation by the tip of the catheter or from perforation of the back wall of the artery by the needle. A retroperitoneal hemorrhage, caused by perforation of the aorta or the pelvic arteries, is particularly treacherous, since it does not usually cause any local symptoms at all. CT-scanning has been described as a useful tool for diagnosing a retroperitoneal hematoma (Illescas et al. 1986).

A *thrombosis* at the place of catheterization mostly causes peripheral ischemia of the involved extremity. After catheterization of the *groin*, the occluded vessel may be either the superficial or the common femoral artery, and the symptoms will vary accordingly. In common femoral artery occlusion (Fig. 3) there is no pulsation in the groin and the peripheral ischemia is severe. In superficial femoral artery occlusion the pulsations are felt in the common femoral artery, but not distally, and the ischemic symptoms are more modest. The thrombus may not always be occlusive (Fig. 2). Spreading of the thrombotic occlusion proximally or distally may alter the clinical picture, sometimes several hours after the catheterization. Basically, the symptoms are characterized by the five P's: pulselessness, paresthesia, paralysis, pain, and paleness.

Emboli to the *lower leg* from catheterization may be large enough to occlude large or medium-sized arteries (Fig. 3) or small enough to enter peripheral vascular branches (Figs. 4, 9). Showers of microemboli may enter the smallest peripheral vessels and, depending on their distribution, cause symptoms of skin rash, livedo reticularis, or "the blue toe syndrome" (Takolander et al. 1985). Catheterization of a severely atherosclerotic aorta may cause massive embolization (Fig. 9) or aortic occlusion (Figs. 5, 10). This complication is sometimes fatal (Takolander et al. 1985).

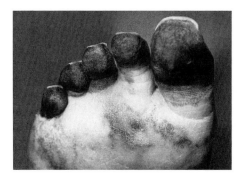

Fig. 9. "Blue toe syndrome" because of microembolization to the healthy leg of a male patient undergoing angiography through the femoral artery because of rest pain in the opposite leg

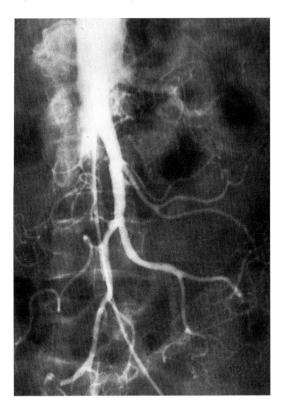

Fig. 10. Aortic occlusion distal to the inferior mesenteric artery due to subintimal catheter dissection during angiography

Arterial occlusion after catheterization of arteries of the *upper extremity* usually causes only mild symptoms due to better collateral circulation. This is true for both brachial and axillary artery occlusions. Loss or weakening of distal pulses are here the most important symptoms. Occasionally, there is paleness and some paresthesia, but rarely paresis or pain. It has been stated repeatedly that these complications often are not diagnosed when the patient is still in the hospital. Some of these patients do, however, later develop symptoms of "arm claudication" when, or if, they go back to work (Bergentz 1987). A few cases of gangrene of fingers or hands have been described (Abrahams 1957). They were probably caused by thromboembolic occlusion spreading distally to the radial and ulnar artery and/or to the finger arteries.

Thromboembolic complications in *arteries other* than the extremity arteries may cause stroke or blindness, myocardial infarction, renal ischemia with infarction or renovascular hypertension, or intestinal infarction (Allen et al. 1965; Andersen 1969; Bergentz et al. 1973; Gill et al. 1972; Takaro et al. 1972; Talner et al. 1975). Most of the thromboembolic complications appear while the patient is still being catheterized or soon after withdrawal of the catheter. Occasionally the complication appears several hours later and, rarely, several days later. This phenomenon may be due to an intimal injury with dissection and thrombosis.

Arteriovenous fistulae after catheterization are mostly of moderate size and rarely cause hemodynamic symptoms (Bolasny and Killen 1971). They are often detected accidentally from a murmur or a thrill in the groin, in the elbow, or over the abdomen. An arteriovenous fistula between the vertebral artery and the vein plexus surrounding this artery causes a murmur which is heard by the patient as a tinnitus (Bergentz et al. 1966; Bergquist 1971; Bergström and Lodin 1966; Björck 1966). Iatrogenic arteriovenous fistulae in infants may become very large, particularly, as described by Ontell and Gauderer (1985) following needle punctures of the radial artery.

A *pseudoaneurysm* can form at the place of catheterization and is felt as an expanding tumor (Fig. 7). It is often difficult to separate this from a small hematoma, which is a normal finding after catheterization and is felt in front of the artery. A pseudoaneurysm is usually a later phenomenon than a hematoma. In contrast to a hematoma, a pseudoaneurysm expands with the pulse wave, which can be felt by bimanual palpation. Furthermore, a machinery murmur can be heard over it.

Prevention

It is impossible to completely avoid complications after such a major diagnostic procedure as an angiography. Several measures can be undertaken, however, in order to decrease the risk (Lang 1967):
1. Angiographies should be performed only in hospitals with a reasonable load of such procedures. It has been demonstrated repeatedly that the number of complications decreases as the number of angiographies carried out in the hospital increases (Adams and Fraser 1973; Hessel et al. 1981).
2. Transfemoral catheterization should be chosen whenever possible (Hessel et al. 1981). In general, catheterization of smaller arteries increases the risk for various types of injury (McMillan and Murie 1984), as does selective catheterization (Rostan and Loup 1978). When arterial catheterization is difficult, or is expected to be difficult, it should be avoided. In these cases, angiographies should be performed using intravenous contrast injection, either with conventional equipment or with digital subtraction angiography (DSA).
3. The time taken for catheterization should be as short as possible, and the catheter should be as thin as possible (Jacobsson and Schlossman 1969).
4. It has been demonstrated that administration of dextran before catheterization decreases the incidence of thrombotic complications without increasing the bleeding (Jacobsson 1969). Heparin given during catheterization also seems to decrease the risk of thromboembolism, but at the same time it increases the incidence of bleeding (Antonovic et al. 1976).

The thrombogenicity of the material used in catheters varies. It has been demonstrated experimentally that if the right catheter material is chosen, the amount of thrombotic material accumulated on the catheter intravascularly decreases (Schlossman 1973; Wilner et al. 1978). No clinical studies are available on the effect of catheter material on the incidence of arterial thromboembolic complications.

Management of the Lesions

Early detection of complications following arterial puncture or catheterization is the key to successful handling. This is particularly important for *thromboembolic occlusions.* A patient who has been undergoing arterial catheterization should be observed, usually for at least 12 h. If the groin has been catheterized, the patient should be in bed during that time. The circulation in the extremities should always be checked by pulse palpation before angiography, immediately after removal of the catheter, and before the patient is allowed to leave the hospital. Oscillography has been suggested as a useful tool for objective assessment of the peripheral circulation, comparing the extremities with each other and comparing the pressure curves before and after catheterization (Jacobsson et al. 1969 b).

Impaired circulation after catheterization is often ascribed to "spasm." Spasm is certainly a problem whenever a catheter is placed in an artery. It has been demonstrated that spasm is more severe if the catheter is wide in relation to the artery (Wickbom and Bartley 1957). This may be one reason why it is more severe in children, in women, and in the upper extremities (Lindbom 1957). Signs of peripheral ischemia persisting for more than a few hours after removal of the catheter should not be ascribed to spasm from the catheterization, however, until arterial thrombi or emboli have been excluded. Confirmation of the diagnosis by a repeated angiography is rarely necessary, at least not in thrombotic lesions at the place of catheter insertion. An angiography may be useful when distal emboli in the extremity are suspected, and necessary when there is suspicion of occlusion of a visceral artery (Jacobsson et al. 1969 b).

When exploring the *femoral* artery for a thrombotic occlusion, bleeding, or pseudoaneurysm after catheterization, it is important to make the skin incision proximal enough to come above the hole which the needle or catheter has made in the artery (Bergentz et al. 1966; Eriksson and Jorulf 1970; Hall 1971; Rutherford and Pearce 1987). This hole is sometimes quite large and lacerated and needs suturing. In these cases it may be easier to remove the thrombus through a separate arteriotomy, rather than through the needle-hole; otherwise, it may be necessary to insert a patch. The use of a Fogarty catheter to clear the distal vascular bed is important. Angiography on the operating table should be used if there is any doubt about whether or not the peripheral vascular bed has been restored to its precatheterization state. The results from early treatment of thromboembolic complications in the lower extremity are practically always satisfactory, the only exception being when microembolization has occurred.

Handling of occlusive injuries of the *brachial* artery after catheterization is more controversial. Some of these patients are asymptomatic in spite of the brachial artery occlusion. It has been pointed out that most of these asymptomatic patients will remain so, particularly if they have restricted activities due to cardiac disease or high age, which often is the case (Bergentz 1988). Other authors have a more active attitude: MacCollum and Mavor (1986) claimed that because of the unpredictability of ischemic symptoms, early exploration and appropriate repair of a brachial artery occlusion should be recommended. However, the results of exploration of the brachial artery and thrombectomy do not seem to be as satisfactory as after thrombectomy of the femoral artery (Bergentz 1988). McCollum and Mavor (1986) report initially successful results in 101 of the 106 brachial arteries explored after occlusion. Forty-five of their patients were treated with resection and reanastomosis, 26 with vein graft interposition, and 25 with thrombectomy and closure. Long-term follow-up studies have not been reported for these patients.

Stroke may be caused by *carotid artery* occlusion from thrombosis or dissection, or from emboli. In the former case, *immediate* exploration and restoration of flow may also restore cerebral function (Bergentz et al. 1966).

Hemorrhage should likewise be handled by early diagnosis and early exploration. One should not wait with the exploration until a large hematoma has developed, as this is almost impossible to evacuate satisfactorily. A retroperitoneal hematoma should be suspected whenever the patient develops signs of unexplained blood loss. Early exploration is mandatory in these cases.

After *carotid artery* puncture it is particularly important to observe the patient closely in order to avoid compression of the larynx and the trachea by a hematoma. Early exploration and tracheotomy are advisable in these cases (Feild and DeSaussure 1965; Helmsoe and Tos 1965). It has also been stressed repeatedly that early exploration is necessary when bleeding is suspected after *axillary artery* catheterization. Molnar and Paul (1972) point out that following removal of the axillary catheter complete hemostasis must be achieved by compressing the proximal portion of the axillary artery for at least 15 min. The patient often experiences some numbness or weakness in the hand, which should disappear within 60 min after completion of the procedure and not return. Persistence of symptoms or development of new symptoms such as tingling, pain, decreased sensation, numbness or weakness in fingers, hand, or arm indicate continued bleeding from the puncture site. In these cases immediate exploration of the axillary artery is mandatory.

Hemorrhage following arterial puncture is usually easy to treat by simple suture. Occasionally, the artery is traumatized to such an extent that a patch is necessary. The hematoma surrounding the arterial perforation should not be approached until the artery has been dissected free and secured above and below.

Most *pseudoaneurysms* are detected one or a few weeks after the catheterization when the hematoma has disappeared, but sometimes not until after several months. Their most common location is in the groin, originating either in the common or the superficial femoral artery. A pseudoaneurysm can probably thrombose and disappear spontaneously, but it can also rupture, and should therefore be operated.

In the surgical treatment of pseudoaneurysm as well, it is important to have control of the artery on each side of the arterial puncture before the pseudoaneurysm is opened. It is then easy to dissect the walls of the pseudoaneurysm free from the artery. The hole in the artery, which by this time usually has smooth edges, will now be seen (Fig. 7). In most cases it is easy to close the hole with one or two longitudinal stiches. Pseudoaneurysms in the axillary artery *are* more difficult to remove surgically but also more important to explore early. Great care has to be taken to avoid injuring the nerve plexus around the axillary artery.

Most *arteriovenous fistulae* are easy to identify and close surgically, or by using a transarterially inserted coil (Keller and Rösch 1985; Nakamura et al. 1985), or by embolization (Mathias 1983). An exception is vertebral arteriovenous fistulae, which are difficult to handle. The entrance of the vertebral artery into the foramen at the 6th transverse process of the cervical vertebra accounts for the relative inaccessibility of this vessel. There is also a great risk of uncontrolled massive hemorrhage from the arterialized vein plexus, the so-called Batson's plexus, surrounding the vertebral artery. Injury to other vital structures, such as the phrenic nerve, the brachial plexus, the pleura, and the cervical cord, during surgery to close a vertebral arteriovenous fistula has been described (Fairman et al. 1984).

The usual technique for closing these fistulae has been exploration of the artery in the vertebral canal below and above the fistula and ligation of the artery at both these places (Bergentz et al. 1966; Bergquist 1971; Bergström and Lodin 1966; Newton and Darroch 1966; Olson et al. 1963). Fairman et al. (1984) described a nonsurgical technique using inflatable balloons in the artery above and below the fistula, or directly occluding the fistula. The success rate with transarterial balloon embolization has been reported to be high (Halbach et al. 1988).

If the patient can tolerate the tinnitus caused by the fistula, the best option seems to be no treatment. Spontaneous closure has also been reported (Bergquist 1971; Newton and Darroch 1966).

References

Abrahams HI (1957) Radiologic aspects of operable heart disease. Radiology 68:812–824

Adams DF, Fraser DB (1973) The complications of coronary arteriography. Circulation 48:609–618

Aguilar S, Kaulbach MG, Hugenholtz PG (1966) Retrograde arterial catheterization of the left ventricle in 388 patients. With special reference to aortic-valve disease and coarctation of the aorta. N Engl J Med 242:312–316

Allen EV (1929) Thromboangitis obliterans: methods of diagnosis of chronic occlusive arterial lesions distal to the wrist with illustrative cases. Am J Med Sci 178:237–244

Allen JH, Parera C, Potts DG (1965) The relation of arterial trauma to complications of cerebral angiography. AJR 95:845–851

Almén T, Boijsen E, Lindell S-E (1977) Metrizamide in angiography. Acta Radiol 18:33–38

Amundsen P, Dietrichson P, Enge I, Williamson R (1963) Cerebral angiography by catheterization – complications and side effects. Acta Radiol 1:164–172

Anagnou J (1982) Cerebrovascular accident during percutaneous cannulation of internal jugular vein. Lancet 2:377–378

Andersen PE (1969) Ischaemic colitis caused by angiography. Clin Radiol 20:414–417

Antonovic R, Rösch J, Dotter CT (1976) The value of systemic arterial heparinization in transfemoral angiography: a prospective study. AJR 127:223–225

Baker WH, Moran JM, Dorner DB (1979) Infected aortic aneurysm following arteriography. J Cardiovasc Surg 20:373–377

Barnes R, Petersen J, Krugmire RB, Strandness E (1978) Complications of brachial artery catheterization: prospective evaluation with the Doppler ultrasonic velocity detector. Chest 66:363–367

Baum V, Eufrate SA (1962) Inferior mesenteric artery injury. A complication of translumbar aortography. NY State J Med 62:3931–3939

Beall AC, Morris GC, Garrett HE et al (1964) Translumbar aortography. Present indications and techniques. Ann Intern Med 60:843–856

Bergentz S-E (1988) Brachial artery occlusions. In: Greenhalgh R (ed) Indications in vascular surgery. Grune and Stratton, London, pp 91–99

Bergentz S-E, Hansson LO, Norbäck B (1966) Surgical management of complications to arterial puncture. Ann Surg 1021–1026

Bergentz S-E, Faarup P, Hegedüs V, Lindholm T, Lindstedt E (1973) Diagnosis of hypertension due to occlusion of a supplemental renal artery: its localization, treatment by removal from the body, microsurgical repair and reimplantation: a case report. Ann Surg 178:643–647

Bergquist E (1971) Bilateral arteriovenous fistulae. A complication of vertebral angiography by direct percutaneous puncture. Two cases, one with spontaneous closure. Br J Radiol 44:519–523

Bergström K, Lodin H (1966) Arteriovenous fistula as a complication of cerebral angiography. Br J Radiol 39:263–266

Björck V-O (1966) Iatrogenic vertebral arteriovenous fistula. Thorax 21:367–368

Blair E, Hunziker R, Flanagan M-E (1970) Catheter embolism. Surgery 67:457–461

Boblitt De, Figley MM, Wolfman EF (1959) Roentgen signs of contrast material dissection of aortic wall in direct aortography. AJR 81:826–834

Bolasny BL, Killen DA (1971) Surgical management of arterial injuries secondary to angiography. Ann Surg 174:962–964

Bouhoutsos J, Morris T (1973) Femoral artery complications after diagnostic procedures. Br Med J 3:396–399

Brodsky JB (1975) Simple method to determine patency of ulnar artery intraoperatively prior to R.A. cannulation. Anesthesiology 42:626–627

Callander CL (1920) Study of arteriovenous fistulae with an analysis of 447 cases. Ann Surg 71:428

Campion BC, Frye RL, Pluth JR, Fairbairn II JF, Davis GD (1971) Arterial complications of retrograde brachial arterial catheterization: a prospective study. Mayo Clin Proc 46:589–592

Cederholm J, Sorensen J, Carlsson C (1986) Thrombosis following percutaneous radial artery cannulation. Acta Anaesthesiol Scand 30:227–230

Chait A, Margulies M (1966) Splenic arteriovenous fistula following percutaneous splenoportography. Radiology 87:518–520

Chiavacci WE, Buciarelli RL, Victorica BE (1976) Aneurysm of the subclavian artery: a complication of retrograde brachial artery catheterization. Cathet Cardiovasc Diagn 2:93–96

Civetta JM, Gabel JC, Gemer M (1972) Internal jugular vein puncture with a margin of safety. Anaesthesia 36:622

Coddon DR, Krieger HP (1958) Circumstances surrounding complications of cerebral angiography. Analysis of 546 consecutive cerebral angiograms. Am J Med 25:580–589

Coran AG, Tyler HB (1968) Aortic dissection. A complication of translumbar aortography. Am J Surg 115:709–711

Crawford ES, Beall AC, Moyer JH, DeBakey ME (1957) Complications of aortography. Surg Gynecol Obstet 104:129–141

Delin A, Fernström I, Swedenborg J (1979) Intimal dissection of the renal artery following selective angiography. Report of two cases and review of the literature. VASA 8:78–82

Downs JB, Rackstein AD, Klein EF, Hawkins IF (1973) Hazards of radial-artery catheterization. Anesthesiology 38:283–286

Dudrick S, Masland W, Mishkin M (1967) Brachial plexus injury following axillary artery puncture. Radiology 88:271–273

Eisenberg RL, Mani RL, McDonald EJ (1976) The complication rate of catheter angiography by direct puncture through aorto-femoral bypass grafts. AJR 126:814–816

Engberg A, Erikson U, Killander A, Persson R, Wicklund H (1974) An usual complication of selective renal angiography. Aust Radiol 18:304–307

Eriksson I, Jorulf H (1970) Surgical complications associated with arterial catheterization. Scand J Thorac Cardiovasc Surg 4:69–75

Fairman RM, Grossman RI, Goldberg HI, Kivuls J, Perloff LJ (1984) A new approach to the treatment of vertebral arteriovenous fistulas. Surgery 95:112–115

Falls HF, Bassett RC, Lamberts AE (1951) Ocular complications encountered in intracranial arteriography. Arch Ophthalmol 45:623–626

Falor WH, Hansel JR, Williams GB (1976) Gangrene of the hand: a complication of radial artery cannulation. J Trauma 16:713–716

Feild JR, DeSaussure RL (1965) Retropharyngeal hemorrhage with respiratory obstruction following arteriography. Case report. J Neurosurg 22:610–611

Feild JR, Lee L, McBurney RF (1972) Complications of 1000 brachial arteriograms. J Neurosurg 36:324–332

Field J, McIvor I, Greenhalgh RM (1987) Transaxillary angiography: an acceptable approach when perfemoral angiography is not acceptable. Eur J Vasc Surg 1:193–195

Fogarty TJ, Krippaehne WW (1965) Vascular occlusion following arterial catheterization. Surg Gynecol Obstet 121:1295–1297

Gill WB, Cole AT, Wong RJ (1972) Renovascular hypertension developing as a complication of selective renal arteriography. J Urol 107:922–924

Gillanders LA (1963) Aortic dissection during translumbar and retrograde abdominal aortography. Br J Radiol 36:725–728

Gudbjerg Ce, Christensen J (1961) Dissection of the aortic wall in retrograde lumbar aortography. Acta Radiol 55:364–368

Guilfoil PH (1963) Inferior-mesenteric-artery syndrome after translumbar aortography. N Engl J Med 269:12–15

Halbach V, Hilashida R, Hieshima G (1988) Treatment of vertebral arteriovenous fistulas. AJR 150:405–412

Hall R (1971) Vascular injuries resulting from arterial puncture or catheterization. Br J Surg 58:513–516

Halpern M (1964) Percutaneous transfemoral arteriography. An analysis of the complications in 1000 consecutive cases. AJR 92:918–934

Hammacher ER, Eikelbom BC, van Tier HIJ, Skotnicki SH, Wijn PFF (1988) Brachial artery lesions after cardiac catheterization. Eur J Vasc Surg 2:145–149

Haney WP, Preston RE (1962) Ocular complications of carotid arteriography in carotid occlusive disease. A report of three cases. Arch Ophthalmol 67:127–137

Harrington JT, Sommers SC, Kassirer JP (1968) Atheromatous emboli with progressive renal failure. Ann Intern Med 68:152–160

Head RM, Robboy SJ (1972) Embolic stroke from mural thrombi, a fatal complication of axillary artery catheterization. Radiology 102:307

Helmsoe L, Tos M (1965) Laryngeal complications of percutaneous cerebral angiography. Acta Otolaryngol (Stockh) 60:175–179

Hessel SJ, Adams DF, Abrams HL (1981) Complications to angiography. Radiology 138:273–281

Illescas FF, Baker ME, McCann R, et al. (1986) CT evaluation or retroperitoneal hemorrhage associated with femoral arteriography. AJR 146:1289–1292

Imoto T, Nobe T, Koga M, Matsukuchi T, Nakata H (1985) Pseudoaneurysm of abdominal aorta: a complication of intrahepatic arterial infusion therapy. J Comput Tomogr 9:279–281

Jacobsson B (1969) Effect of pretreatment with dextran 70 on platelet adhesiveness and thromboembolic complications following percutaneous arterial catheterization. Acta Radiol [Diagn] (Stockh) 8:289–295

Jacobsson B, Schlossman D (1969) Thromboembolism of leg following percutaneous catheterization of femoral artery for angiography. Predisposing factors. Acta Radiol [Diagn] (Stockh) 8:109–118

Jacobsson B, Bergentz SE, Ljungqvist U (1969a) Platelet adhesion and thrombus formation on vascular catheters in dogs. Acta Radiol [Diagn] (Stockh) 8:221–227

Jacobsson B, Paulin S, Schlossman D (1969b) Thromboembolism of leg following percutaneous catheterization of femoral artery for angiography. Symptoms and signs. Acta Radiol [Diagn] (Stockh) 8:97–108

Jonsson K, Lunderquist A, Pettersson H, Sigstedt B (1977) Subintimal injection of contrast medium as a complication of selective abdominal angiography. Acta Radiol [Diagn] (Stockh) 18:55–64

Keller FS, Rösch J (1985) Percutaneous management of iatrogenic arterial-venous fistulas by coil spring occlusion. Eur J Radiol 5:202–205

Kocandrle V, Kittle CF, Petasnick J (1970) Percutaneous retrograde abdominal aortography complication. Intimal dissection. Arch Surg 100:611–612

Lalljee N (1970) Iatrogenic arteriovenous fistula: an unusual complication of cardiac catheterisation. J Cardiovasc Surg 11:246–248

Lang EK (1963) Complications of retrograde percutaneous arteriography. J Urol 90:604–610

Lang EK (1966) Complications of direct and indirect angiography of the brachiocephalic vessels. Acta Radiol [Diagn] (Stockh) 5:296–307

Lang EK (1967) Prevention and treatment of complications following arteriography. Radiology 88:950–956

Lester J (1966) Arteriovenous fistula after percutaneous certebral angiography. Acta Radiol [Diagn] (Stockh) 5:337–340

Lester J, Klee A (1965) Complications of 337 percutaneous vertebral angiographies. Acta Neurol Scand 41:301–314

Lindbom Å (1957) Arterial spasm caused by puncture and catheterization. Acta Radiol 47:449–460

Lindner DW, Hardy WG, Thomas LM, Gurdjian ES (1962) Angiographic complications in patients with cerebrovascular disease. J Neurosurg 19:179–185

Lonni YG, Matsumoto KK, Lecky JW (1969) Postaortographic cholesterol (atheromatous) embolization. Radiology 93:63–65

Mani RL, Eisenberg RL, McDonald EJ, Pollock JA, Mani JR (1978) Complications of catheter cerebral arteriography: analysis of 5000 procedures. I. Criteria and incidence. AJR 131:861–865

Mathias K (1983) Embolisationsbehandlung einer iatrogenen vertebrovenösen Fistel. Fortschr Rontgenstr 138:368–370

Mathieu A, Dalton B, Fischer JE, Kumar A (1973) Expanding aneurysm of the radial artery after frequent puncture. Anesthesiology 38:401–403

McAfee JG (1957) A survey of complications of abdominal aortography. Radiology 68:825–838

McAfee JG, Willson JKV (1956) A review of the complications of translumbar aortography. AJR 75:956–970

McCollum CH, Mavor E (1986) Brachial artery injury after cardiac catheterization. J Vasc Surg 4:355–359

McDowell RFC, Thompson ID (1959) Inferior mesenteric artery occlusion following lumbar aortography. Br J Radiol 32:344–346

McEnany MT, Austen WG (1977) Life-threatening hemorrhage from inadvertent cervical arteriotomy. Ann Thorac Surg 24:233–236

McMillan J, Murie JA (1984) Vascular injury following cardiac catheterization. Br J Surg 71:832–835

Miyasaka K, Edmonds JF, Conn AW (1976) Complications of radial artery lines in the paediatric patient. Can Anaesth Soc J 23:9–14

Molnar W, Paul DJ (1972) Complications of axillary arteriotomies. Radiology 104:269–276

Moore CH, Wolma FJ, Brown RW, Derrick JR (1970) Complications of cardiovascular radiology. A review of 1204 cases. Am J Surg 120:591–593

Nakamura T, Nakashima Y, Yu K, Senda Y et al. (1985) Iatrogenic arteriovenous fistula of the internal mammary artery. Transcatheter intravascular coil occlusion. Arch Intern Med 145:140–141

Neviaser R, Adams J, May G (1976) Complications of arterial puncture in anticoagulated patients. J Bone Joint Surg 58-A:218–220

Newton TH, Darroch J (1966) Vertebral arteriovenous fistula complicating vertebral angiography. Acta Radiol 5:428–440

Olson RW, Baker HL, Svien HJ (1963) Case report and technical note. Arteriovenous fistula: a complication of vertebral angiography. J Neurosurg 20:73–75

Ontell SJ, Gauderer MWL (1985) Iatrogenic arteriovenous fistula after multiple arterial punctures. Pediatrics 76:97–98

Perl S, Wener L, Lyons W (1973) Pseudoaneurysm after angiography. Med Ann D C 42:173–175

Perret G, Nishioka H (1966) Report on the cooperative study of intracranial aneurysms and subarachnoid hemorrhage. Sect. IV. Cerebral angiography. An analysis of the diagnostic valve and complications of carotid and vertebral angiography in 5484 patients. J Neurosurg 25:98–114

Puylaert CBAJ (1965) Fatal and nearly fatal mesenterical infarction, caused by intramural injection in translumbar biphasic aortography. J Belge Radiol 48:671–695

Reiss MD, Bockstein JJ, Bleifer KH (1972) Radiologic aspects of renovascular hypertension. JAMA 221:374–378

Rossi P, Carillo FJ, Alfidi RJ, Ruzicka FF (1974) Iatrogenic arteriovenous fistulas. Radiology 111:47–52

Rostan O, Loup P (1978) Lésions vasculaires iatrogènes. Rev Med Suisse Romande 98:321–327

Rubenson A, Jacobsson B, Sörensen S-E (1979) Treatment and sequelae of angiographic complications in children. J Pediatr Surg 14:154–157

Rutherford RB, Pearce WH (1987) Acute problems following diagnostic and interventional radiological procedures. In: Bergan JJ, Yao JST (eds) Vascular surgical emergencies. Grune and Stratton, New York

Samaan HA (1971) The hazards of radial artery pressure monitoring. J Cardiovasc Surg 12:342–347

Schlossman D (1973) Thrombogenic properties of vascular catheter materials in vivo. The difference between materials. Acta Radiol [Diagn] (Stockh) 14:186–192

Sigstedt B, Lunderquist A (1978) Complications of angiographic examinations. AJR 130:455–460

Slogoff S, Keats AS, Arlund C (1983) On the safety of radial artery cannulation. Anesthesiology 59:42–47

Soderstrom CA, Wassterman DH, Dunham CM, Caplan ES, Cowley RA (1982) Superiority of the femoral artery for monitoring. A prospective study. Am J Surg 144:309–312

Staal A, van Voorthuisen AE, van Dijk LM (1966) Neurological complications following arterial catheterisation by the axillary approach. Br J Radiol 39:115–116

Szilagyi DE, Smith RF, Elliott JP, Hageman JH (1977) Translumbar aortography. A study of its safety and usefulness. Arch Surg 112:399–407

Takaro T, Pifarré R, Wuerflein RD et al. (1972) Acute coronary occlusion following coronary arteriography. Mechanisms and surgical relief. Surgery 72:1018–1029

Takolander R, Bergqvist D, Jonsson K, Karlsson S, Fält K (1985) Fatal thromboembolic complications at aortofemoral angiography. Acta Radiol [Diagn] (Stockh) 26:15–19

Talner LB, McLaughlin AP, Bookstein JJ (1975) Renal artery dissection: a complication of catheter arteriography. Radiology 117:291–295

van Andel GJ (1980) Arterial occlusion following angiography. Br J Radiol 53:747–753

Wagner M (1963) Pseudoaneurysm. A complication of percutaneous angiography and angiocardiography. JAMA 186:427–428

Wickbom I, Bartley O (1957) Arterial „spasm" in peripheral arteriography using the catheter method. Acta Radiol 47:433–448

Wilkins RG (1985) Radial artery cannulation and ischaemic damage: a review. Anaesthesia 40:896–899

Wilner GD, Casarella WJ, Baier R, Fenoglio CM (1978) Thrombogenicity of angiographic catheters. Circ Res 43:424–428

Vascular Injuries from Venous Catheterization

Types of Injury

Venous catheterization may cause four different types of cardiovascular injuries: intravascular foreign body embolism, arterial lesion with bleeding or arteriovenous fistula, perforation of the heart with cardiac tamponade, or venous thromboembolism. The first three types of complication, which may require acute surgical intervention, will be presented in some detail. Venous thromboembolism will be mentioned briefly.

Incidence

Intravascular embolism from pieces of catheters seems to have been relatively common in the 1960s. Pässler et al. (1972) collected 126 cases of catheter embolism from the literature and by inquiry, reviewing about 11 000 cases. In a review, Wellmann et al. (1968) reported on 13 patients who died with catheter embolism. In six of these, catheter embolism was the exclusive or a major contributory cause of death.

Arterial injuries from venous catheterization causing bleeding, arteriovenous fistulae or pseudoaneurysm are probably very rare and known only from case reports. They have been described mainly during the past 10 years, when catheterization of the jugular vein and subclavian vein has been popularized (Farhat et al. 1975; Mills et al. 1986; Nakamura et al. 1985; Ortiz et al. 1979; Wiedemann et al. 1988; Wisheart et al. 1972).

Among 6245 patients who underwent pulmonary artery catheterization with balloon flotation catheters, four cases of pulmonary artery rupture and one case of right ventricle perforation were found (Shah et al. 1984). Paulson et al. (1980) estimated the incidence of pulmonary artery rupture to be much lower, or ten per million users.

Thrombotic complications from indwelling central venous catheters are relatively common, although the number is obviously decreasing, since catheterization through the groin has been abandoned in adults. Efsing et al. (1983) reported an incidence of 12% after catheterization through the subclavian or jugular vein, with the catheter being left in place for between 10 and 13 days. In two of their 159 cases there were clinical signs of pulmonary embolism, including one death. Walters et al. (1972) noted an incidence of asymptomatic thrombosis of about 20%. In an extensive study done at Malmö General Hospital over a 15-year period, Bergqvist and Lindblad (1985) found 41 patients in whom pulmonary embolism was diagnosed at autopsy and originated from a central venous catheter. In seven of these pulmonary embolism was considered to be the cause of death, in 17 to be contributory.

Foreign-Body Embolism Following Venous Catheterization

Causes

There are several reasons for loss of catheter material into the venous system (Bernhardt et al. 1970; Doering et al. 1967; Geraci and Selman 1973; Lewis 1964; Turner and Sommers 1954). In some cases the catheter has broken and dislodged, in others the catheter has accidentally been cut by a needle, particularly at the time when a needle was used as an adapter. Sometimes it is not quite clear what has happened; the catheter has simply disappeared.

At times it has been possible to retrieve the lost catheter material in a peripheral vein (Coblentz 1966). In other cases the catheter has been transported to the superior or inferior vena cava, to the right heart, or to the pulmonary artery (Doering et al. 1967; Friedman and Jurgeleit 1968; Lewis 1964; Taylor and Rutherford 1963; Turner and Sommers 1954). When located in the right atrium or ventricle it may perforate the heart and cause hemopericardium. If the catheter is transported to the pulmonary artery it may sometimes remain there without causing symptoms, or it may cause an (often asymptomatic) pulmonary infarct (Bernhardt et al. 1970). Regardless of the localization, life-threatening sepsis may occur (Doering et al. 1967; Wellmann et al. 1968).

Treatment

The mortality from foreign-body embolism is high. Pässler et al. (1972) found it to be 40% if the foreign body was left intact and 10% after surgical removal.

Several techniques have been described to remove catheter pieces from different parts of the vascular system. Graham et al. (1970) reported six cases, five of them pediatric, in which catheters were removed by open heart surgery using hypothermia (five cases) or bypass surgery. Smyth et al. (1968) described transvenous removal of catheter material from the right atrium by means of an alligator-jawed endoscopic forceps inserted through the external jugular vein. Others (Geraci and Selman 1973; Miller et al. 1970) have described removal of catheters from the heart or from the pulmonary artery using a special snare device. Von Bessler (1977) described the use of a Dormia basket to remove catheters from the superior vena cava and right atrium. Surgical catheter removal may sometimes be necessary after intracardiac knotting of catheters (Lipp et al. 1971).

Arterial Injuries from Venous Catheterization

Arterial injuries from venous catheterization are due to accidental lesion of an artery during insertion of a jugular vein or subclavian vein catheter, or to lesion caused by the tip of the catheter during prolonged cannulation, or lesion of the pulmonary artery from a flow-directed balloon-tipped catheter.

Wisheart et al. (1972) reported an ascending cervical artery lesion with severe hemorrhage, extrathoracic hematoma, and hemothorax following *internal jugular vein catheterization*. Ortiz et al. (1979) reported a lesion of the inferior thyroid artery resulting in an arteriovenous fistula between this artery and the internal jugular vein. Dodson et al. (1980) reported a vertebral arteriovenous fistula after insertion of a catheter in the right jugular vein. McEnany and Austen (1977) reported two cases of life-threatening cervical hemorrhage that occurred during attempts to catheterize the internal jugular vein with a balloon-tipped pulmonary artery catheter in patients heparinized for cardiopulmonary bypass. In one of the patients, two holes in the carotid artery and two in the jugular vein had to be sutured. Several severe complications have been described that occurred following percutaneous puncture and catheterization of the *subclavian vein*. This vein runs adjacent to the subclavian artery but is separated from it by the anterior scalene muscle. The vessels are separated from the thorax only by a thin pleura. Pneumothorax and tension pneumothorax have been the most common complications during insertion of the catheter, but there are also reports of hemothorax from perforation of the back wall of the vein, resulting in leakage of blood into the pleura (Borja 1972; Longerbeam et al. 1965; Matz 1965; Schapira and Stern 1967; Smith et al. 1965). In other cases, there has been perforation of the artery resulting in hemothorax, which may be fatal (Bernhardt et al. 1970), or in formation of a subclavian arteriovenous fistula (Bessler 1977). Vertebral arteriovenous fistula has also been described (Dodson et al. 1980). After prolonged use of indwelling subclavian vein catheters, arteriovenous fistula have occurred between the internal mammary artery and the innominate vein (Nakamura et al. 1985).

In recent years there have been a number of complications from *pulmonary artery catheterization*, some of them requiring surgical intervention. The most serious has been pulmonary hemorrhage from laceration of a small peripheral pulmonary artery. Nonfatal hemoptysis was first described by Lapin and Murray in 1972 and fatal pulmonary hemorrhage in 1973 by Golden et al. A review of 6146 patients was published in 1984 by Shah et al.; severe intrapulmonary hemorrhage occurred in five of them, one of which was fatal. Barash et al. (1981) described six cases of catheter-induced pulmonary artery perforation with severe bleeding. Three of the patients died on the operating table following unsuccessful resuscitative efforts, and a fourth patient died 3.5 weeks after a pneumonectomy. Barash et al. were able to document three different causes of pulmonary artery perforation: eccentric balloon configuration, propelling the balloon through the vessel wall; balloon pressure of 250 mmHg or higher; and tip perforation of the vasculature. Reported cases from the literature are summarized in Table 1. Most of the patients have been female and many of them have been on anticoagulants. Pulmonary artery hypertension obviously increases the risk of perforation because of degenerative changes in the vessel wall.

A pulmonary artery perforation should be suspected whenever there is hemoptysis exceeding 15–30 cc. A "wedge angiogram" will demonstrate extravasation of contrast medium, thereby confirming the diagnosis. A double-lumen endotracheal catheter should be passed to facilitate ventilation and prevent aspiration. Emergency pneumonectomy or lobectomy may be required.

Table 1. Patients with catheter-induced pulmonary artery perforation, reported in the literature

Authors	Age (years)	Sex	Diagnosis	Anticoagulation	Pulmonary artery pressure	Symptoms, signs	Outcome	Comments
Barash et al. (1981)	58	F	Aortic surgery	No	Normal	Hemoptysis	Good	Surgery postponed 3 weeks
	64	M	Heart surgery	No	Increased	Hemoptysis	Good	Surgery postponed 2 weeks
	76	F	Heart surgery	Yes	Increased	Hypotension,	Pneumectomy, death	
	70	F	Coronary surgery	Yes	Increased	Massive hemoptysis	Death	
	74	M	Coronary surgery	Yes	Increased	Massive hemoptysis	Death	
	68	F	Coronary surgery	No	Increased	Massive hemoptysis	Death	
Chun and Ellestad (1971)	39	M	Heart surgery	?	?	Hemoptysis	Good	Surgery postponed 4 days
Golden et al. (1973)	34	F	Heart surgery	Yes	Increased	Massive hemoptysis, pleural blood	Thoracotomy, death	
Lapin and Murray (1972)	59	F	Evaluation of heart failure	Yes?	Increased	Hemoptysis	Good	
Page et al. (1974)	79	F	Post-op. control (abdominal surgery)	?	?	Massive hemoptysis	Death	
Pape et al. (1979)	68	M	Evaluation, valve disease	Yes	Increased	Dyspnea, shock, hemothorax	Death	
	67	F	Myocardial infarction	No	?	Hemoptysis	Death	
	69	F	Heart surgery	Yes	?	Hemoptysis	Death	
	68	F	Evaluation, heart disease	No	Increased	Hemoptysis, hemothorax	Death	

Table 1 (continued)

Authors	Age (years)	Sex	Diagnosis	Anticoagu-lation	Pulmonary artery pressure	Symptoms, signs	Outcome	Comments
Own case	76	F	Aortic surgery	No	?	Hemoptysis	Good	Surgery postponed 3 weeks
Connors et al. (1980)	62	F	Heart surgery	No	Increased		Death post-op.	Lobar hemorrhage
	72	M	Coronary surgery	No	?	Tracheal tube bleeding	Lobectomy, good	Lobar hemorrhage
Paulson et al. (1980)	63	M	Heart surgery	No	?	Hemoptysis	Death	
McDaniel et al. (1981)	75	F	Heart surgery	No	Increased	Tracheal tube bleeding	Good	
	76	M	Heart + coronary surgery	No	Increased	Tracheal tube bleeding	Death	
	67	F	Heart surgery	No	Increased	Tracheal tube bleeding	Lobectomy, good	

Several *prophylactic* measures have been recommended to diminish the risk of intrapulmonary hemorrhage (Pape et al. 1979): the balloon inflation must be done under constant pressure monitoring and must be stopped instantly when the tracing is damped; the catheter tip should be refloated for each wedge-pressure measurement, if possible; the wedge time should be kept to a minimum, particularly in patients with pulmonary hypertension; and fluids should not be used for balloon inflation.

Perforation of the Myocardium with Cardiac Tamponade

Some cases of perforation of the right atrium or ventricle by central venous catheters have been reported (Friedmann and Jurgeleit 1968; Henzel and De-Weese 1971; Johnson 1966; Thomas et al. 1969). The symptom was unexplained hypotension during fluid infusion through a central venous cannula. The hypotension was asssociated with distended neck veins, a quiet precordium, and muffled heart sounds. Several deaths have also been reported (Chabanier et al. 1988; Henzel and DeWeese 1971; Johnson 1966). Immediate pericardiocentesis may be life saving. This should be followed by withdrawal of the catheter to lie with its tip in the vena cava. This complication can be avoided by routinely checking that the tip of the indwelling venous catheter is not in the heart but in the vena cava.

Thromboembolic Complications from Venous Catheterization

The risk of thrombotic complications from venous catheterization increases with the duration of the cannulation. Most of these thrombi are asymptomatic, being detected only with phlebography (Bergqvist and Lindblad 1985; Efsing et al. 1983; Indar 1959; Walters et al. 1972). One of the most important factors contributing to thrombosis is probably the type of catheter material. Efsing et al. (1983) reported that polyethylene catheters caused thrombosis in 20% of cases, as compared with heparinized polyethylene catheters causing thrombosis only in 6%. Teflon material was in between these two, at 9%. Although the majority of the patients are asymptomatic, the risk of pulmonary embolism, even fatal, is real (Bergqvist and Lindblad 1985; Efsing et al. 1983). The problem with sepsis following use of indwelling central venous catheters will not be discussed here.

References

Barash PG, Nardi D, Hammond G, Walker-Smith G, Capuano D et al. (1981) Catheter-induced pulmonary artery perforation. Mechanisms, management, and modifications. J Thorac Cardiovasc Surg 82:5–12

Bessler W (1977) Transvenöse Entfernung embolisierter Katheter. Fortschr Rontgenstr 127:164–167

Bergqvist D, Lindblad B (1985) A 30-year survey of pulmonary embolism verified at autopsy: an analysis of 1274 surgical patients. Br J Surg 72:105–108

Bernhard LC, Wegner GP, Mendenhall JT (1970) Intravenous catheter embolization to the pulmonary artery. Chest 57:329–332

Borja AR (1972) Current status of infraclavicular subclavian vein catheterization. Ann Thorac Surg 13:615–624

Chabanier A, Dany F, Brutus P, Vergnoux H (1988) Iatrogenic cardiac tamponade after central venous catheter. Clin Cardiol 11:91–99

Chun GMH, Ellestad MH (1971) Perforation of the pulmonary artery by a Swan-Ganz catheter. N Engl J Med 284:1041–1042

Coblentz DR (1966) Radiographic detection of plastic catheter embolus. Calif Med 105:357–360

Connors JP, Sandza JG, Shaw RC, Wolff GA, Lombardo JA (1980) Lobar pulmonary hemorrhage. Arch Surg 115:883–885

Dodson T, Quindlen E, Crowell R, McEnany MT (1980) Vertebral arteriovenous fistulas following insertion of central monitoring catheters. Surgery 87:343–346

Doering RB, Stemmer EA, Connolly JE (1967) Complications of indwelling venous catheters. With particular reference to catheter embolus. Am J Surg 114:259–266

Efsing H-O, Lindblad B, Mark J, Wolff T (1983) Thromboembolic complications from central venous catheters: a comparison of three catheter materials. World J Surg 7:419–423

Farhat K, Nakhjavan K, Cope C, Yazdanfar S, Fernadez J et al. (1975) Iatrogenic arterio-venous fistula: a complication of percutaneous subclavian vein puncture. Chest 67:480–482

Fraser R (1987) Catheter-induced pulmonary artery perforation: pathologic and pathogenic features. Hum Pathol 18:1246–1251

Friedman BA, Jurgeleit HC (1968) Perforation of atrium by polyethylene central venous catheter. JAMA 201:1141

Geraci AR, Selman MW (1973) Pulmonary artery catheter emboli: successful nonsurgical removal. Ann Intern Med 78:353–356

Golden MS, Pinder T, Andersson WT, Cheitlin MD (1973) Fatal pulmonary hemorrhage complicating use of a flow-directed balloon-tipped catheter in a patient receiving anticoagulant therapy. Am J Cardiol 32:865–867

Graham KJ, Barratt-Boyes BG, Cole DS (1970) Catheter emboli to the heart and pulmonary artery. Br J Surg 57:184–186

Henzel JH, DeWeese MS (1971) Morbid and mortal complications associated with prolonged central venous cannulation. Awareness, recognition, and prevention. Am J Surg 121:600–605

Indar R (1959) The dangers of indwelling polyethylene cannulae in deep veins. Lancet 1:284–286

Johnson CE (1966) Perforation of right atrium by a polyethylene catheter. JAMA 195:176–178

Krantz EM, Viljoen JF (1979) Haemoptysis following insertion of a Swan-Ganz catheter. Br J Anaesth 51:457–459

Lapin ES, Murray JA (1972) Hemoptysis with flow-directed cardiac catheterization. JAMA 220:1246

Lewis EB (1964) Disappearing plastic cannula. Br Med J 2:1010–1011

Lipp H, O'Donoghue K, Resnekov L (1971) Intracardiac knotting of a flow-directed balloon catheter. N Engl J Med 284:220

Longerbeam JK, Vannix R, Wagner W, Joergenson E (1965) Central venous pressure monitoring. Am J Surg 110:220

Matz R (1965) Complications of determining the central venous pressure. N Engl J Med 273:703

McDaniel DD, Stone JG, Faltas AN, Khambatta HJ, Thys DM et al. (1981) Catheter-induced pulmonary artery hemorrhage. J Thorac Cardiovasc Surg 82:1–4

McEnany MT, Austen WG (1977) Life-threatening hemorrhage from inadvertent cervical arteriotomy. Ann Thorac Surg 24:233–236

Miller RE, Cokerill EM, Helbig H (1970) Percutaneous removal of catheter emboli from the pulmonary arteries. Radiology 94:151–153

Mills J, Miedeman J, Robison J, Hallett J (1986) Minimizing mortality and morbidity from iatrogenic arterial injuries: The need for early recognition and prompt repair. J Vasc Surg 4:22–27

Nakamura T, Nakashima Y, Yu K, Senda Y, Hasegawa O et al. (1985) Iatrogenic arteriovenous fistula of the internal mammary artery. Transcatheter intravascular coil occlusion. Arch Intern Med 145:140–141

Ortiz J, Dean WF, Zumbro GL, Treasure RL (1979) Arteriovenous fistula as a complication of percutaneous internal jugular vein catheterization: case report. Br Med J 141:171

Page DW, Teres D, Harshorn JW (1974) Fatal hemorrhage from Swan-Ganz catheter. N Engl J Med 291:160

Pape LA, Haffajee CI, Markis JE, Ockene IS, Paraskos JA et al. (1979) Fatal pulmonary hemorrhage after use of the flow-directed balloon-tipped catheter. Ann Intern Med 90:344–347

Paulson DM, Scott SM, Sethi GK (1980) Pulmonary hemorrhage associated with balloon flotation catheters. J Thorac Cardiovasc Surg 80:453–458

Pässler HH, Henkemeyer H, Burri C (1972) Gefahren des Kava-Katheterismus. Helv Chir Acta 39:101–105

Schapira M, Stern WZ (1967) Hazards of subclavian vein cannulation for central venous pressure monitoring. JAMA 201:111–113

Shah KB, Rao TLK, Laughlin S, El-Etr AA (1984) A review of pulmonary artery catheterization in 6245 patients. Anesthesiology 61:271–275

Smith BE, Modell JH, Gaub ML, Moya F (1965) Complications of subclavian vein catheterization. Arch Surg 90:228–229

Smyth NPD, Boivin MR, Bacos JM (1968) Transjugular removal of foreign body from the right atrium by endoscopic forceps. J Thorac Cardiovasc Surg 55:594–597

Taylor FW, Rutherford CE (1963) Accidental loss of plastic tube into venous system. Arch Surg 86:177–179

Thomas CS, Carter JW, Lowder SC (1969) Pericardial tamponade from central venous catheters. Arch Surg 98:217–218

Turner DD, Sommers SC (1954) Accidental passage of a polyethylene catheter from cubital vein to right atrium. Report of a fatal case. N Engl J Med 251:844–745

Walters MB, Stanger HAD, Trotem CE (1972) Complications with percutaneous central venous catheters. JAMA 220:1455–1457

Wellmann KF, Reinhard A, Salazar E (1968) Polyethylene catheter embolism. Review of the literature and report of a case with associated fatal tricuspid and systemic candidiasis. Circulation 37:380–392

Wiedeman J, Mills J, Robison J (1988) Special problems after iatrogenic vascular injuries. Surg Gynecol Obstet 166:323–326

Wisheart JD, Hassan MA, Jackson JW (1972) A complication of percutaneous cannulation of the internal jugular vein. Thorax 27:496–499

Vascular Injuries After Percutaneous Transluminal Angioplasty

During the past decade the use of percutaneous transluminal angioplasty (PTA) has become increasingly popular. The results in renal and iliac artery stenosis are, in selected cases, comparable to those with reconstructive surgery, and the method is probably cost-effective (Doubilet and Abrams 1984; Health and Public Policy Committee 1983).

The literature on PTA has been overwhelming during the past few years. Complications are usually not reported in detail, however, and there are relatively few articles dealing exclusively with an analysis of complications in lower extremity and renal PTAs (Beinart et al. 1983; Bergqvist et al. 1987; Castaneda-Zuniga et al. 1984; Connolly et al. 1981; Gardiner et al. 1986; Kuiper et al. 1983; Laerum et al. 1983; Menges et al. 1982; Samson et al. 1984; Schlosser et al. 1979; Seyferth et al. 1983; Richter et al. 1983; Sniderman et al. 1984; Weber and Lübcke 1984; Weilbull et al. 1984; 1987a,b; Zeitler et al. 1982). Many of the vascular injuries that develop in association with PTA are similar to those seen after angiography and other types of catheterization (see p. 8).

Types of Injury

Injuries *at the puncture site* may occur as hemorrhage, pseudoaneurysm, or acute occlusion. Injuries due to *guide-wire and/or catheter manipulation* may take the form of subintimal dissection, spasm, acute occlusion, or arteriovenous fistula. At the *dilatation site* there may be an arterial rupture, a pseudoaneurysm, a balloon rupture, or an occlusion. Finally, there may be distal complications, such as peripheral embolism. Injuries caused by contrast media will not be further discussed in this context, nor will septic complications be analyzed.

Causes of Injury

Complications at Puncture Site

Hematoma at the puncture site after withdrawal of the catheter is a normal consequence of catheterization, although it is usually small and insignificant (Athanasoulis 1980; Laerum et al. 1983; Menges et al. 1982; Sniderman et al. 1984). In the literature on PTA as well as on diagnostic angiographies, small hematomas are usually not reported and the quantitation may be difficult. Hematoma formation is probably more common after PTA than after diagnostic catheterization. One reason is the use of relatively large catheters, up to 9-F. The deflated balloon has a large surface, which is wrinkled and may form sharp edges that can further increase the size of the puncture hole. A ruptured balloon, especially in case of a transverse rupture, widens in an umbrella shape, making it difficult to withdraw from the artery. The Olbert-type catheter causes fewer such problems because the balloon material is closer to the catheter wall at exsufflation and the diameter of the catheter is very little affected by the balloon material. Bleeding may also be caused by transection of collateral branches, not by the puncture hole in the main artery itself (Arfvidsson et al. 1983).

Use of acetylsalicylic acid or other drugs which influence platelet function, and of heparin in connection with the dilatation, may prolong the bleeding time and inhibit the normal coagulation; in combination with a large puncture hole the risk of developing hematoma may be increased because of this impaired hemostasis.

When the posterior wall of the femoral artery is punctured, especially above the inguinal ligament, because of the loose retroperitoneal connective tissue with poor counter pressure there may be large and even fatal hemorrhage (Mahler et al. 1982; Wierny et al. 1974).

In some cases an extravasal hematoma surrounded by organized fibrous tissue liquifies, and a *pseudoaneurysm* is created (Arfvidsson et al. 1983; Johnston et al. 1987; O'Mara et al. 1981; Waltman et al. 1982).

When there is arteriosclerosis at the puncture site, plaque dissection may be the result of the catheterization, leading to the development of an *occlusive thrombus* and subsequent ischemia.

Complications from Guide-Wire and Catheter Manipulation

Subintimal dissection by a guide wire and/or catheter is a common complication, especially in patients with tortuous vessels and extensive arteriosclerosis (Fig. 1).

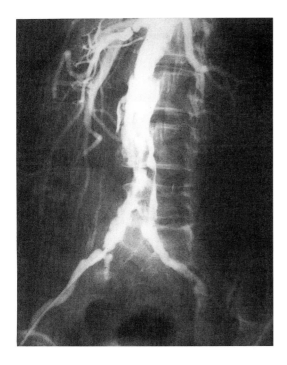

Fig. 1. Subintimal dissection of the aorta following aortic catheterization for dilatation of the renal artery

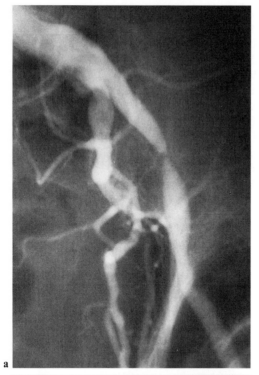

a

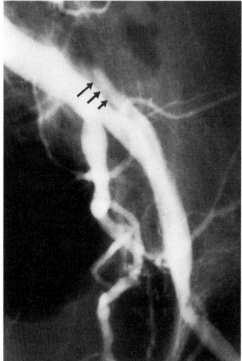

b

Fig. 2. a External iliac stenosis. **b** After successful dilatation there is a dissection proximal to the stenosis (*arrows*)

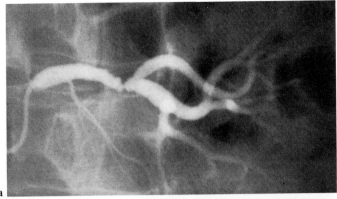

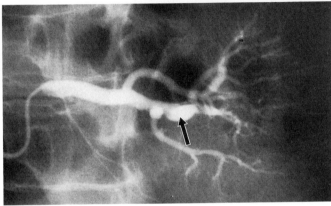

Fig. 3. a Renal artery with fibromuscular dysplasia. **b** After successful dilatation there is a distal subintimal dissection (*arrowhead*) with contrast deposition. There were no clinical manifestations

Thirteen of our procedures (5.5%) were complicated by subintimal dissection (Bergqvist et al. 1987). Usually, the subintimal dissection caused by a guide wire is not harmful (Gardiner et al. 1985). The origin of the dissection is directed distally in the iliac artery, and therefore the blood flow does not usually extend the dissection (Fig. 2). If it is not possible to avoid the dissection track it is advisable to discontinue the procedure and to repeat it later.

In the renal artery a subintimal dissection is a more serious problem (Fig. 3). The origin of the dissection is directed proximally and the dissection may progress in a distal direction to cause total occlusion.

The guide wire or catheter may also penetrate the adventitia, giving rise to hemorrhage and sometimes to an extensive retroperitoneal hematoma. These retroperitoneal hematomas can be diagnosed only by CT and are characterized by back pain. Sometimes the hematoma may extend to the groin and appear several days after the procedure. More rarely, they are so large that they produce hemodynamic effects, necessitating surgical hemostasis.

The manipulation of a guide wire or catheter in an artery may cause a spasm of the catheterized artery, possibly leading to parenchymal damage if it is long-

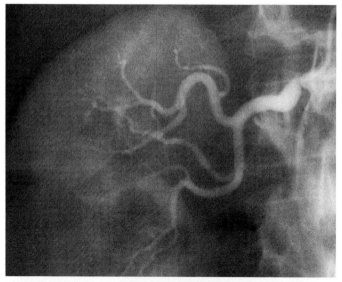

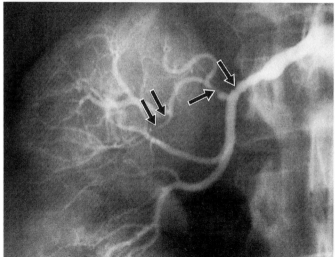

Fig. 4. a Renal artery stenosis. **b** After dilatation there are several spastic segments (*arrowheads*). There were no clinical manifestations

standing (Figs. 4, 5). This usually occurs in the renal arteries and was seen in six patients (5.9%) in our series (Bergqvist et al. 1987). A toxic effect of the contrast medium may contribute to the renal damage. The definition and quantification of spasm may be difficult, and there are no uniform criteria. Beinart et al. (1983) reported a frequency as high as 26% for renal PTAs, and it was much more common in patients with fibromuscular dysplasia than in those with atherosclerosis (46% versus 16%). One possible cause of the postangioplasty vasospasm may be a derangement in arachidonic acid metabolism with a decrease in PGI_2 and PGE_2

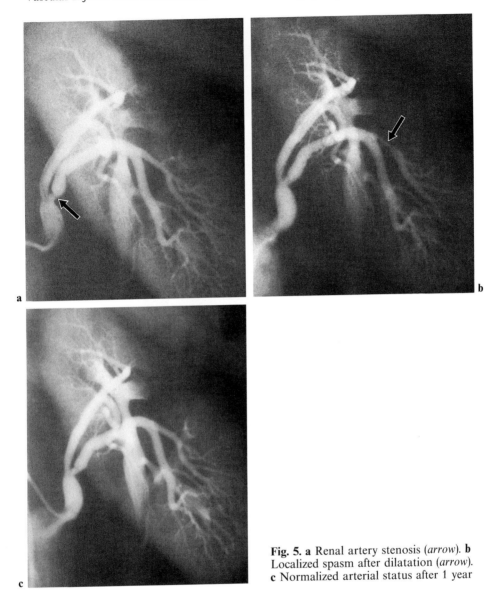

Fig. 5. a Renal artery stenosis (*arrow*). b Localized spasm after dilatation (*arrow*). c Normalized arterial status after 1 year

production and an increase in vasoconstrictor hydroperoxy acids (Cragg et al. 1983).

There were five thrombotic occlusions after our PTA procedures, making an overall frequency of 1.7% (Bergqvist et al. 1987). A fatal case was reported by Takolander et al. (1985). This was a patient who was first dilated because of a left-sided iliac stenosis; the intention was to advance the catheter, turn it around the aortic bifurcation, and advance it down into the right iliac artery for PTA on that side. After this maneuver the aorta occluded, with thrombus progression to the

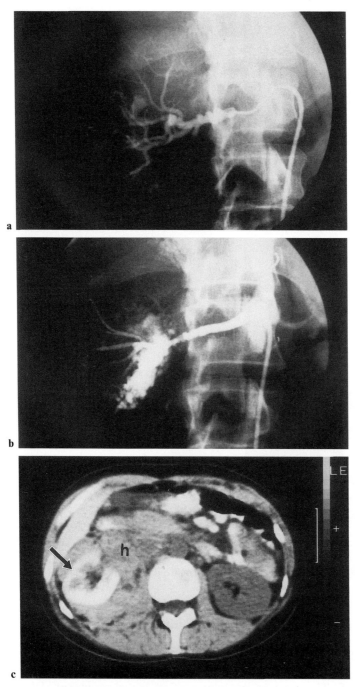

Fig. 6. a Fibromuscular dysplasia in a young female patient. **b** During dilatation the patient developed severe back pain and shock. Extensive contrast extravasation was seen. She improved after conservative treatment. **c** A computerized tomogram shows contrast deposition in the right kidney (*arrow*) and a huge retroperitoneal haematoma (*h*). An exploratory operation was carried out because of recurrent symptoms of active bleeding, and the perforated renal artery was reconstructed

level of the renal arteries. The patient was immediately taken to surgery and a bifurcation graft was inserted. However, there was no backflow whatsoever, the distal vascular bed being totally occluded with widespread necrosis, and the patient subsequently died.

The formation of arteriovenous fistulas secondary to intimal dissection and perforation with a guide wire or catheter has been reported (Lu et al. 1982; Oleaga et al. 1981). These fistulas are usually only temporary and are closed after proper treatment of the stenosis.

Complications at Dilatation Site

Local complications to the dilatation are difficult to foresee. It is important to observe the balloon during dilatation in order to notice any abnormal behavior and distension, indicating a threatening balloon rupture.

Originally, there was a great fear of arterial rupture as a consequence of balloon dilatation. This has proven to be very rare (Berger et al. 1986; Ekelund 1984;

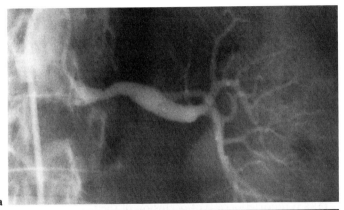

a

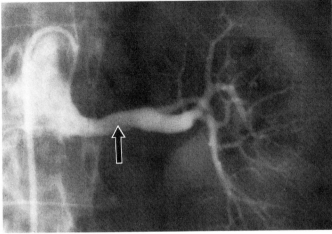

b

Fig. 7. a Renal artery stenosis. **b** After PTA an intimal flap can be seen in the artery (*arrowhead*)

Jensen et al. 1985; Joseph et al. 1987; Lois et al. 1985; Murphy et al. 1987; Richter et al. 1980; Simonetti et al. 1983; Villarica and Gross 1986). Rupture seems to be more frequent after PTA of the renal artery than of other arteries, causing retroperitoneal hematomas, usually self-limiting and characterized by back pain. We had six such patients during renal PTA (5%), and in one surgery was necessary (Fig. 6). Puylaert et al. (1986) reported a delayed renal artery rupture with a fatal outcome. It may be difficult to establish whether the cause is the dilatation or perforation by the catheter or the guide wire. At least in animal experiments, overdistension is a prerequisite for vessel rupture (Zollikofer et al. 1985). Pseudoaneurysm at the dilatation site is a rare but possible complication (Moran and Ruttley 1987).

Balloon rupture during dilatation may cause local damage due to the force with which the contents of the ballon hit the vascular wall. The damage can then be a starting point for a subintimal dissection. We have had six cases (2.5%) in which the balloon ruptured, without causing any sequelae. At the dilatation site, intimal flaps may be seen following dilatation. In our series such flaps were seen in one of the peripheral artery dilatations and in 12 of the renal artery dilatations (Fig. 7). These flaps are usually of no clinical importance; they merely indicate that the dilatation was effective, i.e., that the internal elastic lamina was broken by the balloon (Hoffman et al. 1981).

Occlusion of dilated segments has been reported with a relatively high frequency (Samson et al. 1984). In our series this was seen in three renal arteries, one renal branch artery, and one popliteal artery. In cases of renal artery PTA, complications are seen significantly more often when stenoses are situated close to the aorta (Weibull et al. 1987b; Fig. 8). The location of the stenotic process partly within the aortic wall requires a high dilatation pressure, resulting in more intimal ruptures than with stenoses at other sites. PTA of bifurcation stenosis or of a stenosis close to branches might damage the adjacent artery and cause occlusion through dissection or compression of atherosclerotic material. This is a risk with dilatation of renal artery branch stenoses (Fig. 9).

Catheter trauma to arteries adjacent to the dilated one is also a possibility, although it is rare. Perry (1985) reported a case of occlusion of the superior mesenteric artery as a complication of attempted renal artery PTA.

The mechanism of rapid thrombus formation at the site of dilatation is obscure. In widespread arterial disease, such thrombus formation may be extensive and can cause massive microembolization (Takolander et al. 1985).

Distal Complications

In the beginning of the PTA era there was a great fear of micro- and macroembolism; however, both are seen relatively infrequently. Small asymptomatic or rapidly resolved peripheral emboli probably occur in the majority of PTA procedures, but they very rarely give rise to clinical problems. In an experimental model, Ekelund et al. (1981) found frequent peripheral thromboembolic occlusions with PTA of the renal artery. Dilatation of arteriosclerotic plaques may also cause cholesterol microembolization (Geyskes et al. 1983; Grim et al. 1981). In Figs. 10 and 11 are shown examples of extensive embolic complications.

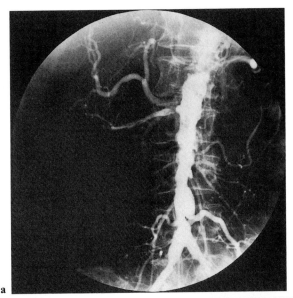

a

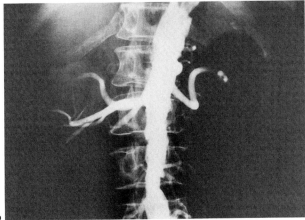

b

Fig. 8. a Severe right-sided renal artery stenosis in a 75-year-old female patient with renovascular uremia, the left renal artery having been occluded for a long time. **b** Successful PTA was performed. **c** After some 12 h the urinary output decreased to almost anuria, a new angiogram showing occlusion (*arrow*), but **d** refilling of the artery after 1 cm (*arrow*). **e** Revascularization with a Dacron patch graft was successful

When a balloon ruptures there is risk that small pieces of the balloon material will embolize; this is often totally asymptomatic, however (Menges et al. 1982).

Incidence

The frequency of the various vessel injuries which may complicate a PTA procedure varies greatly between different series. There may be true differences, but variations are also due to different attitudes toward complications and methods

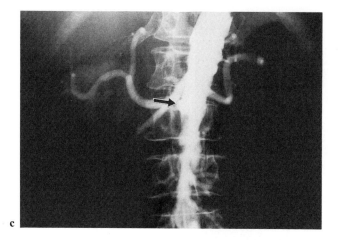

c

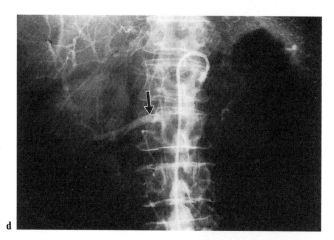

d

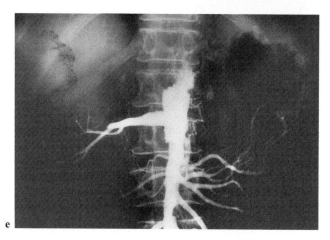

e

Fig. 8. c–e

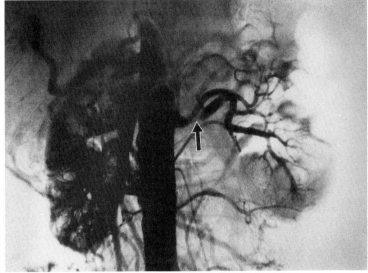

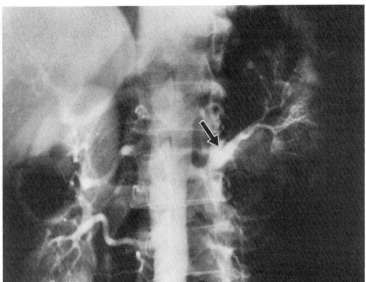

Fig. 9. a Severe stenosis of a branch of the renal artery (*arrow*). **b** After dilatation the nonstenotic branch is occluded (*arrowhead*). Reconstruction with thrombendarterectomy and Dacron patch graft was successful

of registering and reporting them. During the initial period after PTA had been developed as a new therapeutic modality, the beneficial therapeutic effects dominated in publications, and analysis of side effects and complications has developed only gradually. Bergqvist et al. (1987) analyzed 25 recent publications on PTA and found a very depressing picture from the point of view of reporting complications (Table 1). To be able to adequately compare series from different centers, some methodological points must be considered (Bergqvist et al. 1987):

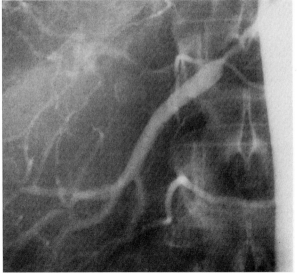

a

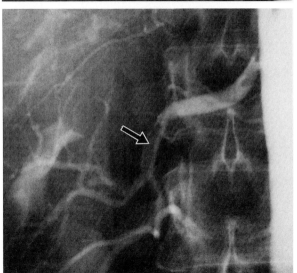

b

Fig. 10. a Renal artery stenosis. **b** After PTA an embolus is located at the first renal artery bifurcation (*arrowhead*)

The *patient material* must be defined in detail, both clinically (sex, age, indication for intervention, symptoms, signs, concomitant diseases) and radiologically (exact localization, length, width, pressure gradient). Inclusion criteria and, equally important, exclusion criteria must be reported.

Technical details as well as the skill and experience of the interventing radiologist must be described. Definition of technical as well as clinical success and failure must be made. When an already published PTA method is referred to all, even small, modifications must be defined. This is also valid for different types of phar-

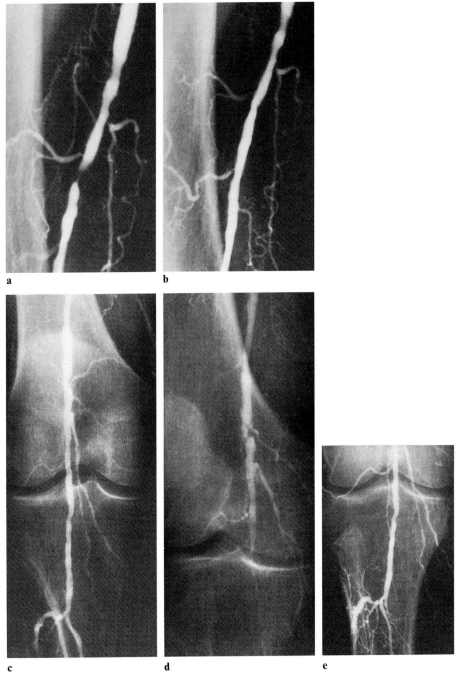

a b c d e

Fig. 11. a Superficial femoral artery stenosis. **b** With PTA the stenosis was successfully treated. **c** The popliteal artery before dilatation. **d** Thromboembolic occlusion of the popliteal artery after PTA of the stenotic superficial femoral artery. **e** The occlusion in the popliteal artery was successfully treated with local infusion of streptokinase

Table 1. How complications are presented in 25 publications (Arfvidsson et al. 1983; Bergqvist et al. 1984; Campbell et al. 1983; Collins et al. 1984; Creutzig et al. 1983; Cumberland 1982; Engel et al. 1982; Fradet et al. 1984; Galichia et al. 1982; Gallino et al. 1982; Glover et al. 1983; Grandt and Madsen 1983; Graor et al. 1984; Haapanen et al. 1984; Jäger et al. 1982; Johnston et al. 1982; Kadir et al. 1983; Knight et al. 1984; Krings et al. 1983; Lu et al. 1982; Pilla et al. 1984; Probst et al. 1983; Rosenørn et al. 1983; Rush et al. 1983; Zeitler et al. 1983)

Complications not defined	25
Frequency of complications given	20
No report on various types of complications	13
Follow-up time for complications given	1
Complications not dealt with in discussion	15

macologic treatment before, during, and after dilatation. The variations in this field are remarkable, and there is no consensus on how to treat these patients pharmacologically (Athanasoulis 1980; Bergentz and Jonsson 1983; Bollinger et al. 1982; Murray et al. 1982; Rusnak et al. 1983; Sos and Sniderman 1981; Zeitler 1979). As we deal with anticoagulants, antiplatelet drugs, and spasm-reducing drugs, different therapeutic regimens may influence the development of bleeding as well as thrombotic complications. The most common practice is to give heparin during the PTA procedure, but doses vary between 2000 and 10 000 IU. Some investigators start antiplatelet treatment a few days before PTA, others do not use it at all. After the dilatation the variations are even greater, in both the short and the long term. With renal PTA, some authors use agents to reduce postdilatory spasm, while others do not. To stress this problem further, Table 2 shows data from 25 reports listed in *Index Medicus* for 1983 and 1984 dealing with lower-extremity PTA. Of the 25 reports, six (24%) did not give any information on how the patients were treated pharmacologically. For the long-term course there are three methods of treatment: no treatment at all, oral anticoagulation, or various types and combinations of antiplatelet drugs. Finally, when some form of pharmacologic treatment is used, doses and durations vary greatly.

Complications must be defined. The scientifically most proper way is to define complications before PTA and then to analyze their number and consequences prospectively. As we have just emphasized, it is important to distinguish between complications occurring at the puncture site and those occurring at the dilatation site, as well as between distal and general complications. It is also necessary to distinguish complications with real clinical implications from those which cause only minimal discomfort and those which are seen only radiographically.

Thus, comparison between studies is connected with a great deal of uncertainty as to what the incidence of complication really means. Weibull et al. (1987b) surveyed ten publications on 675 renal procedures. Major complications

Table 2. Summary of 25 studies concerning pharmacologic treatment against occlusion in connection to and after PTA (see Table 1)

Drug treatment	No. of studies	Drug treatment	No. of studies
Before PTA		Long-term treatment	
No treatment	4	No treatment	2
Not stated	16	Not stated	10
ASA	1	ASA	3
ASA + dipyridamole	3	ASA + dipyridamole	3
Other	1	Anticoagulants	2
During PTA		Different methods and	5
No treatment	1	combinations	5
Not stated	8	Duration of treatment (months)	
Heparin	15	Not stated	15
Other	1	<3 months	2
Immediately after PTA		3–6 months	3
Not stated	16	>6 months	3
Heparin	4	No treatment	2
Dextran	5		

were reported in 3.1%–15.4% and minor ones in 2.2%–30.8%. With an increasing number of publications there is no indication that a lower frequency of complications is reported. In a recent series, Cambria et al. (1987) encountered 20% of cases with complications, 8.5% of which were considered major. Technical complications detected with radiology have only rarely been mentioned, but Weibull et al. (1987a) suggested that they may be important to report because, although asymptomatic, they indicate the risk of development of more severe injuries. Such injuries with dissection, intimal flaps, and small thrombi and emboli may in fact be considered part of the PTA procedure with intimal and plaque fracturing (Block et al. 1980). In a recent series the incidence of vascular complications leading to surgery was similar in patients undergoing transfemoral cardiac catheterization and transfemoral PTA (Skillman et al. 1988).

Tables 3 and 4 show complications that occurred in various series of peripheral and renal artery PTA. The frequency of complications after PTA of an extremity (Table 3) varies considerably between 2.8% and 40.7%, which leads to the suspicion of marked differences in definitions and in reporting routines. There is almost the same degree of variation in the frequency of complications leading to surgical correction, 0.8%–8%. Criteria for surgical correction of a complication are also somewhat arbitrary, however. Increased experience – from 384 PTA (Johnston and Colapinto 1982) to 984 (Johnston et al. 1987) – did not change the frequency of complications; if anything, there was a slight increase. The most common complication is, not surprisingly, minor groin hematoma, in 2.7% (0% –20%) of cases, whereas groin hemorrhage necessitating surgery occurs in only 0.2% of cases. A similar pattern is seen after renal artery PTA. In our series of renal artery PTAs (Weibull et al. 1987) there were significantly more complications in female than in male patients. One reason might be that patients with fi-

Table 3. Survey of complications after PTA of iliac and femoropopliteal arteries

Complications	Arfvidsson et al. (1983)	Campbell et al. (1983)	Colapinto (1986)	Collins et al. (1984)	Creutzig et al. (1983)	Engel et al. (1982)	Eri and Gjølberg (1985)	Freimann et al. (1981)	Galichia et al. (1982)	Gallino et al. (1982)	Glover et al.(1983)	Grandt and Madsen (1983)
No. of patients	51	33	59	100	80	32	134		47	205	83	60
No. of procedures	54	40	64	124	80	32	161	208	66	250	83	95
Major												
Occlusion main artery	2	2						4	1			
Distal embolization		1	2	1	23	2	10	2	1	5	5	2
Retroperitoneal bleeding									1			
Groin hematoma (op.)	1						4	3				1
Pseudoaneurysm, groin (op.)	1						1					
Intimal damage, groin (op.)												
Balloon rupture (op.)												
Brachialis plex. lesion												
Laceration of artery					2							
Minor												
Groin hematoma					1	3	1	6		8	12	2
Guide-wire perforation			2									2
Spasm										1		1
Punction												
Radiologically detected subintimal dissection, arteriovenous fistula, or puncture site thrombosis	1									8	10	2
Surgery necessary												
No. of patients	4	3	1	2	4	2	7	–	1	6	2	
Percentage	7.4	7.5	1.6	1.6	5	6.3	4.3	–	1.5	2.4	2.4	
Complications/procedure (%)	9.3	7.5	6.3	3.2	38.8	9.4	11.8		3.4	3.0	8.8	34.9

bromuscular dysplasia often are young women with reactive vessels more prone to spasm. Another possible explanation is that female arteries are more narrow, which makes manipulation with guide wires and catheters more difficult.

Prevention

Just as in angiography, meticulous technique is important to avoid as many complications as possible. One way to avoid at least unnecessary complications is to keep the indications for PTA very strict. PTA is a valuable tool in our therapeutic armamentarium against arterial diseases, but there must always be close cooperation between the vascular surgeon who establishes the indications and the interventional radiologist who performs the procedure. Moreover, it is a fastidious technique which requires experience and cannot be left to unexperienced col-

Graor et al. (1984)	Johnston et al. (1987)	Kadir et al. (1983)	Knight et al. (1984)	Krings et al. (1983)	Krepel et al. (1985)	Nelzén et al. (1985)	Romianiuk et al. (1987)	Rosenørn et al. (1983)	Rush et al. (1983)	Schneider et al. (1982)	Spangen et al. (1983)	Waltman et al. (1982)	Weibull et al. (1987a)	Total	% of total procedures
58	902	112			129	28	887	31	86		23	160	127		
60	984	141	91	1129	164	30	860	31	97	882	25	198	134	6083	
	15		9	9	2	1	21	2				4	4	76	1.2
2	6	2	1	10	4	2	16		1			2	2	102	1.7
				2										1	
1	1			1							1	2		14	
	1													7	
1														1	
														2	
	51	8	18	16	3				7	25			4	165	2.7
			9				20	3	2					38	0.7
					1									3	
		2												2	
	6			7		3	20	1					10	66	1.1
	1													3	
l	11	2	3	–		2	2	14	–	2	22	2	8	2	105	1.7
.7	1.1	1.4	3.3	–		1.2	6.7	1.6	–	2.1	2.5	8	4.8	1.9	1.7
i.7	9.5	8.5	40.7		33.3	6.1	26.7	9.0	19.4	10.3	2.8	8	4.0	14.9	7.9

leagues. There must be strict and well-defined indications to perform PTA, and it must never be done as a radiologic cosmetic procedure. It is furthermore important to perform PTA only where vascular surgical expertise is available, should complications requiring an urgent operation occur. Although no controlled trials exist, it is probably advisable to use some kind of antibiotic prophylaxis similar to what is used during vascular surgical procedures. The patients should be treated as surgical patients with operating room-like sterility.

The catheter used should be as thin as possible while still providing for adequate dilatation. The femoral artery must be entered below the inguinal ligament to avoid retroperitoneal hematoma. Occasionally, punctures above the inguinal ligament cause this complication, especially when the posterior wall of the artery is punctured several centimeters proximal to the anterior wall puncture due to an obliquely directed needle. Posterior wall puncture should be avoided if at all possible. Careful compression and frequent checking of the puncture site, the ipsilat-

Table 4. Survey of complications after PTA of renal arteries

Complications	Colapinto (1986)	Geyskes et al. (1983)	Grim et al. (1981)	Hägg et al. (1985)	Madias et al. (1981)	Mahler (1982)	Martin et al. (1986)	Miller et al. (1985)	Schwarten et al. (190)	Sos and Sniderman (1981)	Tegtmeyer and Beziudjian (1981)	Waltman et al. (1982)	Weibull et al. (1987b)	Total	% of total procedures
No. of patients	80	70	26	12		16	200	63		89	166	37	101	1078	
No. of procedures		70	26	12	13	19	301	71	78	104					
Major															
Occlusion main artery	3				2		11	2			2	1	4	25	2.3
Distal embolization		12	1			1		1			3		2	20	1.9
Retroperitoneal bleeding					1				1				2	4	0.4
Groin hematoma (op.)							4		2	3			1	10	0.9
Pseudoaneurysm, groin (op.)															
Intimal damage groin (op.)															
Balloon rupture (op.)										1				1	0.1
Laceration of artery															
Minor															
Groin hematoma	2						3						4	9	0.8
Guide-wire perforation							1							1	0.1
Spasm															
Radiologically detected subintimal dissection or arteriovenous fistula		7		2		1				5			14	29	2.7?
Surgery necessary															
No. of patients	3	–	–	–	–	1	5	2	3	4	2	–	5	25	2.3
Percentage	3.8					6.3	1.7	3.2	3.8	3.8	1.2		5	2.3	
Complications/procedure (%)	6.3	27.1	3.8	16.5	23.0	12.5	6.3	4.2	3.8	8.7	3.0	2.7	26.7		

eral leg, and the general condition of the patient after the procedure are important. During the procedure the guide wire should be kept in the catheter, and if small corrections of the catheter position have to be made during the procedure, the catheter will follow the guide wire to minimize the risk of intimal damage by the tip of the catheter. This is especially important when the Olbert type of balloon catheter is used, where the tip of the catheter is movable and moves distally at the evacuation of the balloon catheter. The use of introduction sheaths at the puncture site has proven to be of limited value, as the exsufflated balloon material usually does not pass through the sheath. The Olbert catheter may, however, be introduced and pulled out through a sheath. Subintimal dissection is often avoided by the use of a J-shaped guide wire, which does not penetrate the vessel wall as easily as a straight guide wire.

When a guide wire is introduced into the renal artery it is preferable to have the tip of the guide wire as far out as possible to reach a stable position and to minimize the risk of guide-wire dislocation by the balloon catheter. If the tip of the straight guide wire is put too far out there is a risk of perforation and bleeding in the parenchyma, or of causing a subcapsular and perirenal hematoma (Ekelund 1984). Many authors therefore use a J-shaped guide wire to avoid this kind of complication, but, in our experience, it is easier to reach a stable position with a straight guide wire rather than with a J-guide wire. When serious arterial complications of renal PTA occur there must always be a possibility to solve the problem surgically. The primary aim should be renal revascularization, but a nephrectomy must be considered in situations where the injury makes repair of the artery and the parenchyma impossible.

The catheter must always be turned downwards in the aorta on the contralateral side with utmost care, and if the bifurcation is arteriosclerotic this should preferably be avoided. One possible complication is dissection with aortic occlusion, which is serious and possibly fatal (Takolander et al. 1985). When a spasm occurs, intra-arterial injection of lidocaine-papaverine, nitroglycerin, or calcium blockers such as verapamil and nifedipine has been recommended, and the treatment is usually effective (Lu et al. 1982; Sos and Sniderman 1981). Avoiding spasm is an even more attractive alternative, and this is possible with lidocaine and tolazoline, and α-blocker (Beinart et al. 1983). The use of calcium antagonists has also been recommended (Beinart et al. 1983; Sos and Sniderman 1981), because of their effect during coronary artery PTA (Kaltenbach et al. 1982).

When performing the dilatation it is probably important to have correct balloon pressure and to be aware of the possibility of obtaining very high pressure by manual force.

Treatment

When complications which require surgical intervention do occur, the therapeutic options really do not differ much from those available after complications of angiography and cardiac catheterization (see p. 8). Microembolization of atherosclerotic debris or thrombotic material is often difficult to treat. The emboli lodged in larger vessels can usually be removed by embolectomy. When this is not possible, another option is to locally infuse low-dose streptokinase or urokinase into the affected artery. Several dose regimens have been suggested; in our hands, the infusion of 5000 units of streptokinase per hour has been successful. For obvious reasons, this will work only on material that is of true thrombotic origin and not on atherosclerotic material or cholesterol crystals. Another source of embolism is a ruptured balloon, which, however, often remains asymptomatic (Menges et al. 1982); if not, an embolectomy must be tried.

In some cases external compression is not sufficient to stop the bleeding at the puncture site, making surgical hemostasis necessary. In these cases it is important to mobilize the whole artery, making proximal and distal control possible as well as providing the opportunity to inspect the whole vessel circumference. Sometimes an arteriotomy must be performed to stop the bleeding. The Seldinger technique with an oblique puncture makes the perforations in the adventitia, media, and intima on separate levels and the bloodstream may cause a subintimal dissection. If there is a puncture hole in the back wall it is more proximal than the hole in the front wall.

In cases of vessel rupture it is important to keep the balloon catheter in place and, by inflating the balloon at the rupture site, to prevent unnecessary bleeding from the rupture hole. The artery is then rapidly exposed and reconstructed according to the situation. In some cases it may be sufficient to temporarily tamponade the laceration with the balloon to obtain adequate and continued hemostasis (Joseph et al. 1987).

A method for retrieving a ruptured balloon catheter through a sheath has been reported (Tegtmeyer and Bezirdjian 1981).

References

Arfvidsson B, Davidsen JP, Petersson B, Spangen L (1983) Percutaneous transluminal angioplasty (PTA) for lower-extremity arterial insufficiency. Preliminary results of two years' applications. Acta Chir Scand 149:43–47

Athanasoulis C (1980) Percutaneous transluminal angioplasty. General principles. AJR 135:893–900

Beinart C, Sos T, Saddekni S, Weiner M, Sniderman K (1983) Arterial spasm during renal angioplasty. Radiology 149:97–100

Bergentz S-E, Jonsson K (1983) Percutaneous transluminal angioplasty. A review. Acta Chir Scand 149:641–649

Berger T, Sörensen R, Konrad J (1986) Aortic rupture. A complication of transluminal angioplasty. AJR 146:373

Bergqvist D, Takolander R, Jonsson K, Karlsson S, Hellekant C (1984) Percutaneous transluminal angioplasty of arteriosclerotic lesions in the pelvis and lower extremities. Acta Chir Scand 150:445–449

Bergqvist D, Jonsson K, Weibull H (1987) Complications after percutaneous transluminal angioplasty of peripheral and renal arteries. A review article. Acta Radiol [Diagn] (Stockh) 28:3–12

Block P, Fallon J, Elmer D (1980) Experimental angioplasty: lessons from the laboratory. AJR 135:907–912

Bollinger A, Schneider E, Kuhlmann U, Pouliadis G, Brunner U (1982) Percutaneous transluminal angioplasty (PTA). State of the art and future perspectives. Vasa 11:369–370

Cambria R, Faust G, Gusberg R, Tilson D, Zucker K, Modlin I (1987) Percutaneous angioplasty for peripheral arterial occlusive disease. Arch Surg 122:283–287

Campbell WB, Jeans WD, Cole SEA, Baired RN (1983) Percutaneous transluminal angioplasty for lower-limb ischaemia. Br J Surg 70:736–739

Castaneda-Zuniga W, Tadavarthy M, Laerum F, Amplatz K (1984) "Pseudo"-intramural injection following percutaneous transluminal angioplasty. Cardiovasc Intervent Radiol 7:104

Colapinto R, Stronell R, Johnston W (1986) Transluminal angioplasty of complete iliac obstructions. AJR 146:859–862

Collins RH, Voorhees AB, Reemtsma K, Todd GJ, Hardy MA, Nowygrod R (1984) Efficacy of percutaneous angioplasty in lower-extremity arterial occlusive disease. J Cardiovasc Surg 25:390–394

Connolly J, Kwaan J, McCart M (1981) Complications after percutaneous transluminal angioplasty. Am J Surg 142:60

Cragg A, Einzig S, Castaneda-Zuniga W, Amplatz K, White J, Rao G (1983) Vessel wall arachidonate metabolism after angioplasty: possible mediators of postangioplasty vasospasm. Am J Cardiol 51:1441–1445

Creutzig A, Luska G, Elgeti H, Alexander K (1983) Perkutane Angioplastie der unteren Extremitäten im fortgeschrittenen Lebensalter. Dtsch Med Wochenschr 108:1543–1546

Cumberland DC (1982) Percutaneous angioplasty in complete iliac occlusions. Vasa 11:297–300

Doubilet P, Abrams HL (1984) The cost of underutilization. Percutaneous transluminal angioplasty for peripheral vascular disease. N Engl J Med 310:95–102

Ekelund L (1984) Increased kidney size following renal angioplasty. A "new" observation. Acta Radiol [Diagn] (Stockh) 25:401–405

Ekelund L, Jonsson N, Lindstedt E, Stridbeck H, Lundquist S-E (1981) Dilatation of experimental renal artery stenosis by balloon catheter. Acta Radiol [Diagn] (Stockh) 22:561–569

Engel A, Adler OB, Rosenberger A (1982) Percutaneous transluminal angioplasty of the iliac and lower-limb vessels. Isr J Med Sci 18:921–927

Eri LM, Gjølberg TØ (1985) Percutaneous transluminal angioplasty in the lower extremities (in Norwegian). Tidsskr Nor Laegeforen 105:503–506

Fradet G, Lidstone D, Herba M, Chiu RJC, Blundell PE (1984) Percutaneous transluminal angioplasty of iliac arteries. The importance of functional studies. Can J Surg 27:359–361

Freimann DB, Spence RK, Gatenby R (1981) Transluminal angioplasty of the iliac and femoral arteries: follow-up results without anticoagulation. Radiology 141:347–350

Galichia JP, Duick GF, Bajaj AK, Roberts RW (1982) Percutaneous transluminal angioplasty. The treatment of stenotic or occluded iliac arteries. J Kans Med Soc 83:553–557

Gallino A, Mahler F, Probst P, Nachbur B (1982) Früh- und Spätergebnisse bei 250 perkutanen transluminalen Dilatationen an den unteren Extremitäten. Vasa 11:319–321

Gardiner GA, Meyerovitz MF, Harrington DP et al. (1985) Dissection complicating angioplasty. AJR 145:627

Gardiner G, Meyerovitz M, Stokes K, Clouse M, Harrington D, Bettmann M (1986) Complications of transluminal angioplasty. Radiology 159:201–208

Geyskes GG, Puylaert CBAJ, Oei HY, Mees D (1983) Follow-up study of 70 patients with renal artery stenosis treated by percutaneous transluminal dilatation. Br Med J 287:333–336

Glover JL, Bendick PJ, Dilley RS, Becker GJ (1983) Balloon catheter dilation for limb salvage. Arch Surg 118:557–560

Grandt M, Madsen B (1983) Early results of percutaneous transluminal angioplasty (in Danish). Ugeskr Laeger 145:1670–1672

Graor RA, Young JR, McCandless M et al. (1984) Percutaneous transluminal angioplasty. Review of iliac and femoral dilatations at the Cleveland Clinic. Cleve Clin Q 51:149–154

Grim CE, Luft FC, Yunek HY, Klatte EC, Weinberger MH (1981) Percutaneous transluminal dilatation in the treatment of renal vascular hypertension. Ann Intern Med 95:439–442

Haapanen A, Keski-Nisula L, Ala-Ketola L (1984) Percutaneous dilatation of lower-leg arteries. Ann Clin Res [Suppl 16] 40:7–9

Health and Public Policy Committee, American College of Physicians (1983) Percutaneous transluminal angioplasty. Ann Intern Med 99:864

Hoffman MA, Fallon JT, Greenfield AJ, Waltman AC, Athanasoulis CA, Block PC (1981) Arterial pathology after percutaneous transluminal angioplasty. AJR 137:147

Hägg A, Lörelius L-E, Mörlin C, Åberg H (1985) Percutaneous transluminal renal artery dilatation for fibromuscular dysplasia with special reference to the acute effects on the renin-angiotensin-aldosterone system and blood pressure. Scand J Urol Nephrol 19:205–209

Jäger K, Schneider E, Grüntzig A, Bollinger A (1982) Perkutane transluminale Angioplastie (PTA) im frühen Stadium II der peripheren arteriellen Verschlußkrankheit. Vasa 11:332–335

Jensen SR, Voegeli DR, Crummy AB, Turnispeed WD, Acher CW, Goodson S (1985) Iliac artery rupture during transluminal angioplasty. Treatment by embolization and surgical bypass. AJR 145:381–382

Johnston KW, Colapinto RF (1982) Peripheral arterial transluminal dilatation. Early results. Can J Surg 25:532–534

Johnston W, Rae M, Hogg-Johnston S et al. (1987) Five-year results of a prospective study of percutaneous transluminal angioplasty. Ann Surg 206:403–413

Joseph N, Levy E, Lipman S (1987) Angioplasty-related iliac artery rupture: treatment by temporary balloon occlusion. Cardiovasc Intervent Radiol 10:276–279

Kadir S, Hill-Zobel RL, Tsan MF (1983) Evaluation of arterial injury due to balloon angioplasty by ^{111}In-labelled platelets. Nucl Med 22:324–328

Kaltenbach M, Kober G, Scherer D (1982) Transluminal coronary angioplasty and intracoronary thrombosis. Transbrachial approach and prevention of thromboembolic complications. In: Kaltenbach M, Grüntzig A, Rentrop K, Bussman WD (eds) Coronary heart disease, part IV. Springer, Berlin Heidelberg New York, p 23

Knight RW, Kenney GJ, Lewis EE, Johnston GG (1984) Percutaneous transluminal angioplasty. Am J Surg 147:578–582

Krepel VM, van Andel GJ, van Erp WFM, Breslau PJ (1985) Percutaneous transluminal angioplasty of the femoropopliteal artery: initial and long-term results. Radiology 156:325–328

Krings W, Roth FJ, Rieger H (1983) Früh- und Spätergebnisse der perkutanen transluminalen Angioplastie von Beckenarterienstenosen. Med Welt 34:773–774

Kuiper KJ, de Jong PE, Zeeuw D, Schuur KH, van der Hem GK (1983) Restenosis of the renal artery after percutaneous transluminal renal angioplasty. An inevitable outcome? Proc Eur Dial Transplant Assoc 20:538

Laerum F, Castaneda-Zuniga WR, Amplatz KA (1983) Complications of transluminal angioplasty. In: Castaneda-Zuniga WR (ed) Transluminal angioplasty. Thieme, New York, p 41

Lois JF, Takiff H, Schechter MS, Gomes AS, Machleder HI (1985) Vessel rupture by balloon catheters complicating chronic steroid therapy. AJR 144:1073–1074

Lu CT, Zarins CK, Yang CF, Turcotte JK (1982) Percutaneous transluminal angioplasty for limb salvage. Radiology 142:337–342

Madias NE, Ball JT, Millan VG (1981) Percutaneous transluminal renal angioplasty in the treatment of unilateral atherosclerotic renovascular hypertension. Am J Med 70:1078–1084

Mahler F, Probst P, Haertel M, Weidmann P, Krneta A (1982) Lasting improvement of renal hypertension by transluminal dilatation of atherosclerotic and nonatherosclerotic renal artery stenoses. A follow-up study. Circulation 65:611–617

Martin L, Casarella W, Alspaugh J, Chuang V (1986) Renal artery angioplasty: increased technical success and decreased complications in the second 100 patients. Radiology 159:631–634

Menges HW, Altstaedt F, Bayer P, Storz LW, Hoevels J (1982) Art und Häufigkeit PTA-induzierter Komplikationen und ihre Bedeutung für Notfallchirurgie. Vasa 11:274

Miller GA, Ford KK, Braun SD, Newman GE et al. (1985) Percutaneous transluminal angioplasty vs. surgery for renovascular hypertension. AJR 144:447–450

Moran CG, Ruttley MST (1987) Development of false aneuryms following percutaneous transluminal angioplaty. Br J Surg 74:652

Murray P, Garnic D, Beitmann M (1982) Pharmacology of angioplasty and intravascular thrombolysis. AJR 139:795–803

Murphy T, Cronan J, Paolella L, Dorfman G, Francis W (1987) Arterial rupture without balloon rupture during percutaneous transluminal angioplasty. J Vasc Surg 6:528–530

Nelzén O, Berglund G, Brunes L, Hallböök T (1985) PTA is an acceptable complement to vascular surgery (in Swedish). Läkartidningen 82:3058–3059

Oleaga JA, Grossman RA, McLean GK, Rosen RJ, Freimann DB, Ring EJ (1981) Arteriovenous fistula of a segmental renal artery branch as a complication of percutaneous angioplasty. AJR 136:988

O'Mara CS, Neiman HL, Flinn WR, Herman RJ, Yao JST, Bergan JJ (1981) Hemodynamic assessment of transluminal angioplasty for lower-extremity ischemia. Surgery 89:106–117

Perry M (1985) Intermural dissection of superior mesenteric artery. A complication of attempted renal artery balloon dilation. J Vasc Surg 2:480–484

Pilla TJ, Peterson GJ, Tantana S, Lang ER, Wolverson MK (1984) Percutaneous recanalization of iliac artery occlusions. An alternative to surgery in the high-risk patient. AJR 143:313–316

Probst P, Cerny P, Owens A, Mahler F (1983) Patency after femoral angioplasty. Correlation of angiographic appearance with clinical findings. AJR 140:1227–1232

Puylaert CBAJ, Mali WRTM, Rosenbusch G, van Straalen AM, Klinge J, Feldberg MAM (1986) Delayed rupture of renal artery after renal percutaneous transluminal angioplasty. Radiology 159:635–637

Richter EI, Grüntzig A, Ingrisch H (1980) Percutaneous dilatation of renal artery stenoses. Ann Radiol (Paris) 23:275

Richter EI, Krönert E, Zeitler E (1983) Technique, indications, complications, and results of percutaneous transluminal renal artery dilatation. In: Dotter CT, Grüntzig AR, Schoop W, Zeitler E (eds) Percutaneous transluminal angioplasty. Springer, Berlin Heidelberg New York, p 286

Romaniuk P, Wierny L, Münster W (1987) Long-term effectiveness of angioplasty versus operation in iliac and femoropopliteal obstructions. In: Oeser H (ed) Angiological symposium, Berlin, pp 39–49

Rosenørn MA, Harling OJ, Hegedüs V, Hesse B, Høilund-Carlsen PF (1983) Percutaneous transluminal angioplasty for arterial insufficiency of the lower extremities (in Danish). Ugeskr Laeger 145:1673–1677

Rush DS, Gewertz BL, Lu CT, Ball DG, Zarins CK (1983) Limb salvage in poor-risk patients using transluminal angioplasty. Arch Surg 118:1209

Rusnak B, Castaneda-Zuniga W, Amplatz K (1983) The use of anticoagulants in transluminal angioplasty. In: Castaneda-Zuniga W (ed) Transluminal angioplasty. Thieme, New York

Samson RH, Sprayregen S, Veith FJ, Scher LA, Gupta SK, Ascer E (1984) Management of angioplasty complications, unsuccessful procedures and early and late failures. Ann Surg 199:234

Schlosser V, Spillner G, Mathias K (1979) Komplikationen nach perkutaner transluminaler Gefässrekanalisation (PTR) und ihre chirurgische Behandlung. Vasa 8:324

Schneider E, Grüntzig A, Bollinger A (1982) Langzeitergebnisse nach perkutaner transluminaler Angioplastie (PTA) bei 882 konsekutiven Patienten mit iliakalen und femoropoplitealen Obstruktionen. Vasa 11:322–326

Schwarten De, Yune HY, Klotte EC, Grim CE, Weinberger MH (1980) Clinical experience with percutanous transluminal angioplasty (PTA) of stenotic renal arteries. Radiology 135:601–604

Seyferth W, Ernsting M, Grosse-Vorholt R, Zeitler E (1983) Complications during and after percutaneous transluminal angioplasty. In: Dotter CT, Grüntzig AR, Schoop W, Zeitler E (eds) Percutaneous tranlsuminal angioplasty. Springer, Berlin Heidelberg New York, p 161

Simonetti G, Rossi P, Passariello R et al. (1983) Iliac artery rupture. A complication of transluminal angioplasty. AJR 140:989–990

Skillman J, Kim D, Baim D (1988) Vascular complications of percutaneous femoral cardiac interventions. Incidence and operative repair. Arch Surg 123:1207–1212

Sniderman K, Bodner L, Saddekni S, Srur M, Sos T (1984) Percutaneous embolectomy by transcatheter aspiration. Radiology 150:357–361

Sos TA, Sniderman KW (1981) Percutaneous transluminal angioplasty. Semin Roentgenol 16:26–41

Spangen L, Persson B, Arfvidsson B, Davidsen JP (1983) PTA – one alternative for patients with a leg threatened with amputation (in Swedish). Läkartidningen 80:4023–4024

Takolander R, Bergqvist D, Jonsson K, Karlsson S, Fält K (1985) Fatal thrombo-embolic complications at aorto-femoral angiography. Acta Radiol [Diagn] (Stockh) 26:15–19

Tegtmeyer CJ, Bezirdjian DR (1981) Removing the stuck, ruptured angioplasty balloon catheter. Radiology 139:231

Villarica J, Gross R (1986) Treatment of angioplasty-related iliac artery rupture without bypass surgery (case report). AJR 147:389-390

Waltman AC, Greenfield AJ, Novelline RA et al. (1982) Transluminal angioplasty of the iliac and femoropopliteal arteries. Arch Surg 117:1218–1221

Weber J, Lübcke P (1984) Combined PTA and low-dose transcatheter fibrinolysis in PTA-induced complications and arterial thrombosis. Ann Radiol 27:334

Weibull H, Törnquist C, Bergqvist D et al. (1984) Reversible renal insufficiency after percutaneous transluminal angioplasty (PTA) of renal artery stenosis. Acta Chir Scand 150:295

Weibull H, Bergqvist D, Jonsson K, Carlsson S, Takolander R (1987a) Complications after percutaneous transluminal angioplasty in the iliac and femoro-popliteal arteries. J Vasc Surg 5:681–686

Weibull H, Bergqvist D, Jonsson K, Carlsson S, Takolander R (1987b) Analysis of complications after percutaneous transluminal angioplasty of renal artery stenoses. Eur J Vasc Surg 1:77–84

Wierny L, Plass R, Postmann W (1974) Long-term results in 100 consecutive patients treated by transluminal angioplasty. Radiology 112:542–548

Zeitler E (1978) Drug treatment before and after percutaneous transluminal recanalization (PTR). In: Zeitler E (ed) Percutaneous vascular recanalization. Springer, Berlin Heidelberg New York, pp 73–77

Zeitler E, Ernsting M, Richter EI, Seyferth W (1982) Komplikationen nach PTA femoraler and iliakaler Obstruktionen. Vasa 11:270

Zeitler E, Richter EI, Roth FJ, Schoop W (1983) Results of percutaneous transluminal angioplasty. Radiology 146:57

Zollikofer CL, Salomonowitz E, Castaneda-Zuniga WR, Bruhlmann WF, Amplatz K (1985) The relation between arterial and balloon rupture in experimental angioplasty. AJR 144:777–779

Radiation-induced Vascular Injuries

Types of Injury

Radiation-induced vascular injuries can manifest themselves as stenosis and thrombotic or fibrotic occlusion, aneurysm, dilatation, or rupture. A special situation of rupture is the development of a fistula into the gastrointestinal tract, a so-called secondary arterioenteric fistula (Bansky et al. 1984; Bergqvist 1987; Estrada et al. 1983; Georgelin et al. 1973; Kwon et al. 1978; Vetto et al. 1987). This has also been reported as a duodenocaval fistula (Rheudasil et al. 1988).

Special Problems Concerning Vascular Radiation Injury

It has been known for several decades that various types of radiation can induce microscopic as well as macroscopic alterations in vessels. Unfortunately, many of the histological alterations are rather unspecific and mimic the atherosclerotic process, and in some cases there is an acceleration of the development of arteriosclerosis as the main effect of radiation. The process is slow, which means that many patients with a malignant disease do not live long enough to develop the full clinical picture of radiation-induced vascular damage. For these reasons, it has been difficult to establish a cause relationship.

Factors Indicating Radiation-induced Injury

1. Vessel injuries are seen within the radiation field (Budin et al. 1976; Guthaner and Schmitz 1982; Servo and Puranen 1978).
2. There are healthy vessels within other parts of the organism (Budin et al. 1976; Colquhoun 1966; Guthaner and Schmitz 1982; Hughes et al. 1984; Liegl 1975; McReynolds et al. 1976; Ormerod 1976; Painter et al. 1975; Rosenfeld et al. 1987; Thomas and Forbus 1959; Wright and Bresnan 1976). Patients with radiation-induced carotid artery injury had less evidence of generalized atherosclerotic disease than did control patients, as indicated by angiography (Silverberg et al. 1978).
3. Localization of the process is atypical compared with that of atherosclerosis. Radiation injury is often localized in the distal part of subclavian artery, whereas atherosclerosis is usually localized to the proximal part (Budin et al. 1976; Fig. 1). Carotid arteriosclerosis is most frequently localized to the bifurcation whereas radiation-induced injury often is seen proximally in the com-

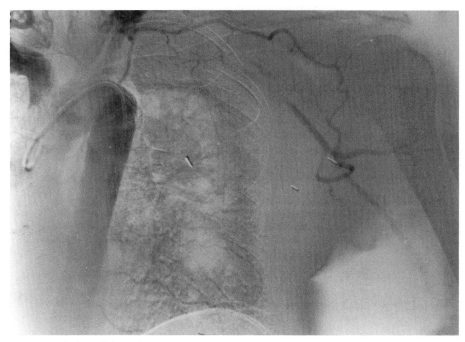

Fig. 1. Occlusion of the subclavian artery in a non-smoking 82-year-old female, undergoing irradiation because of mammary cancer 5 years previously. The occlusion is localized more distally than what is typical for atherosclerosis

mon carotid artery (Eisenberg et al. 1978; Guthaner and Schmitz 1982; Hayward 1972; Levinson et al. 1973; Nardelli et al. 1978; Pepin et al. 1976; Silverberg et al. 1978; Fig. 2).
4. Radiation injury to adjacent tissue such as skin, subcutaneous tissue, muscles, skeleton, lungs, intestines, kidneys, bladder, or thyroid gland is seen (Butler et al. 1980; Dibbell and Gowen 1965; Gross et al. 1969; Hegarty et al. 1969; Johnson let al. 1969; Joseph and Shumrick 1973; Kretschmer et al. 1986; Levinson et al. 1973; Mavor et al. 1973; McCall et al. 1959; McCready et al. 1983; McReynolds et al. 1976; Reiter et al. 1979; Rotman et al. 1969; Servo and Puranen 1978).
5. The patients are younger than those who develop arteriosclerosis (Butler et al. 1980; Cohn et al. 1967; Conomy and Kellermeyer 1975; Darmody et al. 1967; Dollinger et al. 1966; Fraumeni et al. 1967; Georgelin et al. 1973; McCready et al. 1983; McEniery et al. 1987; McGill et al. 1979; McReynolds et al. 1976; Nardelli et al. 1978; Painter et al. 1975; Poulias et al. 1967; Servo and Puranen 1978; Staab et al. 1976; Thomas and Forbus 1959; Wright and Bresnan 1976). Silverberg et al. (1978) found that radiated patients with atherosclerotic occlusive disease in the carotid arteries were 10 years younger on average than control patients. As an example of the difficulty with age may be mentioned

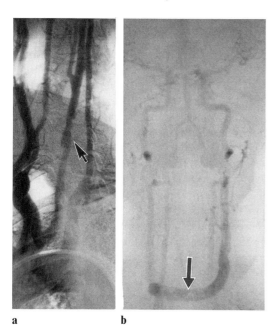

Fig. 2. a Female patient, irradiated 20 years previously because of a malignant tumour in the larynx. Frequent transitory ischemic attacks indicated angiography, which showed irregular atherosclerosis-like formations in the common carotid artery (*arrows*). b Reconstruction was carried out using ligation of the common carotid artery and a Dacron crossover graft from the other side (*arrow*). Microscopy showed advanced atherosclerotic alterations with fibrosis

a   b

the case described by Fehér (1965): A 69-year-old man received radiation therapy because of lung cancer. Three weeks later he developed myocardial infarction, and the author felt that there was probably a cause relationship. As the patient was at the age where arteriosclerotic complications are common, this was very difficult to prove.

6. The histological picture is typical for radiation-induced fibrosis with endothelial proliferation (Darmody et al. 1967; Dollinger et al. 1966; Nardelli et al. 1978).
7. The amount of irradiation has exceeded accepted safe levels (Darmody et al. 1967; McReynolds et al. 1976; Staab et al. 1976).
8. The patient has no or few known risk factors for the development of arteriosclerosis (McEniery et al. 1987; McReynolds et al. 1976). McEniery et al. (1987) compared risk factors in patients with coronary artery disease who had or had not undergone previous radiation therapy. The irradiated patients were significantly less often males and smokers and significantly less often hypercholesterolemic.

Vascular reaction to Radiation

Initially after radiation, some authors have reported segmental contractions which can be reversed by intra-arterial papaverine (Bosniak et al. 1969; Hopewell 1974). Fonkalsrud et al. (1977) made scanning electron micrographs of radiated dog femoral arteries. After 48 h there were extensive surface changes with severe nuclear distruption, accompanied by extensive crater formation. After 1 week there were no normal cells and minimal deposition of fibrin and platelets. After 3 weeks there was a sporadic resurfacing of the intima with short plump cells without the normal spatial order. After 6 weeks, sparsely placed elongated cells were seen but not a normal endothelium. After 4 months the reparative process had progressed with spindle-shaped cells, but there were still cell fragments and craters with irregular edges. By and by, the intima becomes markedly proliferated and fibrotic, with luminal reduction and eventually occlusion (Budin et al. 1976; Fraumeni et al. 1967; Gross et al. 1969; Hatcher et al. 1985; Hopewell 1980; Lindsay et al. 1962; Poon et al. 1968; Sheehan 1944). In the regions of intimal hyperplasia there may also be development of arteriosclerotic-like plaques (Lindsy et al. 1962) with calcification (Nardelli et al. 1978). Painter et al. (1975) described arteriosclerosis out of proportion in the radiated zone but relatively normal vessels within other localizations. There may also be fibromuscular proliferation without signs of atheromatosis (Fajardo and Lee 1975; Dollinger et al. 1966). The internal elastic membrane is also injured with thickening and fraying, disruption and fragmentation (Budin et al. 1976; Heidenberg et al. 1966; Johnson et al. 1969; Lindsay et al. 1962; Marcial-Rojas and Castro 1962; Poon et al. 1968; Sams 1965; Savlov et al. 1969; Sheehan 1944), and sometimes it is not even visualized (Nardelli et al. 1978). Subintimal edema is seen (Marcial-Rojas and Castro 1962). The collagen and smooth-muscle fibers are often preserved (Poon et al. 1968) and, at least in mice, an increased production of collagen with a sort of hyaline thickening has been reported (Sams 1965). Hyalinized vessels with narrowing of lumina have also been described in radiated patients (Rubin et al. 1963). The adventitial tissue undergoes fibrosis with focal hemorrhage and infiltration of lymphocytes (Budin et al. 1976; McReynolds et al. 1976; Nardelli et al. 1978; Poulias et al. 1967; Thomas and Forbus 1959). Using yttrium 90 for pituitary ablation, Kaufman et al. (1966) described extensive alterations within the internal carotid artery related to the area of radiation: the smooth-muscle cells were destroyed, the media being converted into a hyalinized, anuclear layer with coagulation necrosis and fragmented irregularly shaped cells without nuclei. In a patient with Hodgkin's disease Kagan et al. (1971) described a characteristic picture of a foam-cell-like arteritis within the radiated field. Foam cell development has also been described in experimental situations in rabbits, especially in hyperlipemic animals (Kirkpatrick 1967; Konings et al. 1975). Rupture is preferentially seen in elastic vessels, with very little calcification but with myointimal proliferation and extensive necrosis in the adventitial tissue (Fajardo and Lee 1975). There are several experimental studies indicating a potentiating effect between hypercholesterolemia and radiation for the development of atheromatous plaques (Aarnoudse and Lamberts 1977, Amromin et al. 1964; Gold 1961; Konings et al. 1975; Lamberts and de Boer 1963). Silverberg et al. (1978) provided data from a clinical series supporting this observation. In rats, at least, there are data showing that hypertension accelerates vascular damage after cerebral irradiation (Hopewell et al. 1970).

Radiation of rat arteries and veins induces diminished fibrinolytic activity over time as measured histochemically (Åstedt et al. 1974). The synthesis of prostacyclin (PGI_2) as measured with radioimmunologic assay increases immediately after radiation, with a subsequent decrease over the following days to levels well below the starting values (Sinzinger et al. 1983). Cells close to the lumen are preferentially activated in acid phosphatase, while the media contains more β-glucuronidase-activated cells, thus indicating an activation of lyzosomal enzymes (Konings et al. 1975). There is also a depolymerization of vessel wall mucopolysaccharides, resulting in atheromatosis (Aarnoudse and Lamberts 1977).

Butler et al. (1980) described the influence of time on the types of injuries seen clinically as follows:
1. Injuries developing within 5 years consisted of mural thrombi.
2. Injuries seen at about 10 years were of the fibrotic-occlusion type.
3. Injuries late in the course (mean 26 years) consisted of periarterial fibrosis combined with an accelerated arteriosclerotic process.

The time lapse to rupture is mostly much shorter than the stenotic, symptom-producing process. Among 177 patients reported in the literature considered to have radiation-induced arterial disease, 63% had an occlusive process, 35% rupture or erosion, and 2% aneurysm. The median time until stenotic symptoms occurred was 11 years (9 months–52 years); time until rupture was considerably shorter, or 6 months (10 days–10 years). In seven of the 177 cases radiation was given for benign diseases: cutaneous hemangiomas in three (McCready et al. 1983; Poulias et al. 1967; Wright and Bresnan 1976), hyperthyreoidism in two (Hayward 1972; Levinson et al. 1973) and benign lymph-node swelling in the neck (von Krückemeyer 1973) and tonsillitis (Rotman et al. 1969) in one each. All developed stenotic lesions, but with a very long delay, the median time being 32 years with a range of 6–52.

Incidence

The incidence of radiation-induced vascular injuries is largely unknown. One obvious difficulty is the long time it takes to develop an injury giving rise to clinical symptoms and signs, which presents problems in establishing a cause relationship. Another difficulty is the pathologic and also angiographic similarity between radiation-induced injury and arteriosclerosis; sometimes it is perhaps just a somewhat accelerated arteriosclerotic process. The third difficulty is the lack of prospective studies in which a radiated population is followed over time. A fourth difficulty has to do with the increased mortality due to the malignant process, allowing no time for the clinical picture of radiation injury to become overt.

Annest et al. (1983) found four patients who had been mediastinally radiated among 558 patients who had undergone coronary bypass in the period 1978–1982. They extended their study, investigating 163 patients who had received irradiation for Hodgkin's disease, non-Hodgkin's lymphoma, and thymoma. Among the 74 who had been radiated more than 10 years previously, there was an 18% prevalence of major coronary events, which by far exceeded the expected risk based on data from the Framingham study. Elerding et al. (1981) did a retrospective study of 910 patients with head and neck radiation and a survival of more than 5 years. They looked for patients with a fixed neurologic deficit (>24 h) and

found 63 patients (6.3%) who had had a cerebral infarction, 12 of whom underwent reconstructive extracranial carotid surgery. Their mean age was 64 years,
and the mean interval between radiation and infarction was 9 years (1.5–18).
Compared with a control population, the expected number of patients was 38
($P = 0.39$). The same authors also did a study on 300 similar patients, starting with
a questionnaire. One hundred and eighteen responded; they had also undergone
carotid phonoangiography (CPA), oculoplethysmography (OPG), and periorbi-
tal directional Doppler investigation. Fourteen patients (12%) had symptoms.
CPA was abnormal in 17 of 77 investigations (22%). Twenty had abnormal OPG.
The total incidence of abnormalities found on these investigations was 25%, of
which 8% were hemodynamically insignificant.

Glicksman and Nickson (1973) did a study of early and late radiation reactions after treatment for Hodgkin's disease. They mentioned a Takayasu-like aor-
titis as a rare complication but did not discuss vessel involvement beyond that.
Joseph and Shumrick (1973) investigated 173 consecutive patients with surgery
head and neck cancer. The patients were divided into three groups: (a) those
without radiation, 46 patients; (b) those with planned radiation of 4000–4500 R
during 3–4 weeks with the delay of surgery for 4–5 weeks, 35 patients;
(c) unplanned radiation. They had received either curative radiation or previous
preoperative radiation and surgery, radiation of at least 4000 R, 22 patients.
The frequency of necrosis of the carotid artery was 0%, 28%, and 50% respectively, that of mortality due to complications 0%, 0%, and 36% respectively.

Risk Factors

Several risk factors have been mentioned as important:
1. Overlap between subsequent radiation fields (Benson 1973)
2. Repeated series of radiation therapy with a dose beyond demonstrated
   tolerance (Benson 1973; Darmody et al. 1967; Loeffler 1975)
3. Large single total dose (Fajardo and Lee 1975; Iqbal et al. 1977; McReynolds
   et al. 1976)
4. A combination of surgery and radiation within the same anatomic area (Borsanyi 1962; Deppe et al. 1984; Joseph and Shumrick 1973; Marcial-Rojas and
   Castro 1962; McCall et al. 1959; McCready et al. 1983; Vetto et al. 1987)
   In cases of rupture, more risk factors have been discussed:
1. The surgical procedure and complications of this procedure, such as loss of
   skin flaps, wound infection, tissue necrosis (Deppe et al. 1984; Dibbell et al.
   1965; Fajardo and Lee 1975; Hegarty et al. 1969; Joseph and Shumrick 1973;
   Ketcham and Hoye 1965; Kretschmer et al. 1986; Marcial-Rojas and Castro
   1962; McCall et al. 1959; McCready et al. 1983; Poon et al. 1968; Roscher et
   al. 1966)
2. The development of salivary fistula, considered a high risk factor in cases of
   head and neck malignancy (Dibbell et al. 1965; Marcial-Rojas and Castro
   1962; McCall et al. 1959; McConnell and Marlowe 1972; McCready et al.
   1983). In one reported case an orocutaneous fistula had eroded the hyoid

bone, the sharp fragment puncturing the carotid artery, with exsanguination (McConnell and Marlowe 1972).

3. Recurrence of the malignant process (Dibbell et al. 1965; Fajardo and Lee 1975).

4. Since the intestine is more sensitive than the arteries to radiation, it has been suggested that high-dose radiation may lead to bowel necrosis and sepsis, and to subsequent erosion of arteries and development of an arterioenteric fistula (Kinsella and Bloomer 1980; Vetto et al. 1987).

   However, Fajardo and Lee (1975) made an analysis of factors in cases of large artery rupture, and their conclusion was somewhat contradictory to that of others mentioned above. They considered radiation to be not the only cause and perhaps not even the most important one:

1. Surgery has been performed in most patients who have skin flap slough, infection, fistula formation, where salivary fistulas are considered especially dangerous because of protease activity with damage to the adventitial tissue.

2. Morphological analysis suggested damage secondary to perivascular inflammation.

3. In rare cases, rupture may occur without radiation.

4. If radiation were the most important or the sole factor, more of this type of complication after radiation of the mediastinum would have been reported.

5. While the incidence of rupture appears to increase proportional to the extent of the surgical procedure, there is no indication that the incidence may increase with the radiation dose.

Angiographic Findings

Dencker et al. (1972) investigated patients who had been radiated within the pelvis and had had intestinal complications. Angiographically, there were occlusions and tortuous vasa recta, and the distribution of alterations within the bowel were irregular. In places of bowel stricture there were occluded arteries and arteriovenous shunting.

Long irregular stenoses and ulcerations, and sometimes occlusions with atypical localization compared with the arteriosclerotic process, are considered indicative of radiation-induced injury (Eisenberg et al. 1978; Levinson et al. 1973; Nardelli et al. 1978; Pepin et al. 1976; Poulias et al. 1967). Heidenberg et al. (1966) described a Takayasu-like picture of the aortic arch and proximal vessels.

The finding of a pseudoaneurysm or an aneurysm under an ulcerated part of the skin is considered typical (Kretschmer et al. 1986).

Von Breit (1969) performed angiography of around 70 gynecologic patients before and after radiation therapy. The investigated vessels were divided into those more than 8 mm, those less than 8 mm, and those less than 2 mm. The author found size-related changes after radiation, but there was a possibility of different radiation doses to vessels of different sizes, and therefore the conclusion may not be perfectly valid. In any case, there was narrowing of all vessels and arteriosclerosis in the larger ones.

Clinical Picture

The first report of radiation-induced large-vessel injury was given by Thomas and Forbus (1959). The alterations were seen in the aortic arch of a patient radiated for a mediastinal lymphoma.

Patients with radiation-induced injuries very often have radiation damage of other tissues in the vicinity. The symptom development is otherwise typical for the involved vessel and in that respect does not deviate from the pictures seen in cases of occlusive arteriosclerosis. In addition to ischemic disease of the leg and arm arteries, there have been reports of renovascular hypertension (Crummy et al. 1965; Gerlock et al. 1977; Lee et al. 1976; McGill et al. 1979; Staab et al. 1976), myocardial infarction (Cohn et al. 1967; Dollinger et al. 1966; Huff and Sanders 1972; Iqbal et al. 1977; McEniery et al. 1987; Rasmussen et al. 1978; St. Louis et al. 1974; Tracy et al. 1974), transient ischemic attacks, stroke, or amaurosis fugax (Bergqvist et al. 1986; Eisenberg et al. 1978; Glick 1972; Hayward 1972; Kagan et al. 1971; Levinson et al. 1973; Liegl 1975; Nardelli et al. 1978; Rotman et al. 1969; St Louis et al. 1974; Von Krückemeyer 1973; Wright and Bresnan 1976), hemiparesis because of occlusion of the medial cerebral artery (Darmody et al. 1967), intestinal ischemia (McGill et al. 1979), and pulseless (Takayasu's) disease (Heidenberg et al. 1966). The by far predominating arteries with stenotic radiation injuries are the carotid artery, the iliac artery, and the subclavian artery.

Stenotic occlusive disease usually progresses slowly; much more dramatic are cases with rupture and hemorrhage. This bleeding can be external (Fajardo and Lee 1975), subcutaneous, into the gastrointestinal tract as an arterioenteric fistula, or, as in one case, in the form of a tracheoinnominate artery fistula (Reiter et al. 1979). In this last case there was no surgery or no tracheal cannula but an advanced radiation fibrosis with a tracheal stenosis. The carotid artery is the most common with rupture (approximately 77% of all ruptures). In patients with arterioenteric fistulas the dominating symptom is severe gastrointestinal hemorrhage (Bansky et al. 1984; Bergqvist 1987; Estrada et al. 1983; Georgelin et al. 1973; Kwon et al. 1978; Vetto et al. 1987), and none of the hitherto reported cases have survived. The four aneurysms reported were located in the subclavian (Kretschmer et al. 1986), common femoral (Hegarty et al. 1969; Ross and Sales 1972), and deep femoral arteries (Benson 1973).

When surgery is performed within radiation-injured areas, anatomic landmarks may be destroyed and there may also be difficulties in defining adequate anatomic dissection planes. This may therefore lead to laceration of large vessels, with heavy hemorrhage as the result.

Prevention and Therapy

One difficult situation is when there is a combination of radiation and surgery in the head and neck region, where there is a high risk of carotid artery rupture and of exsanguinating hemorrhage. The risk can probably be minimized by rotating tissue flaps to cover the devitalized and necrotizing areas (Conley 1953). Meticulous surgical technique is important to avoid wound complications. Neck incisions close and parallel to the carotid arteries should be avoided, since breakdown of such wounds will expose the vessel.

When there is an abundance of necrotic tissue adjacent to the vessels, a prophylactic ligation with extra-anatomic bypass must be considered. An example of this is the use of an obturatory bypass to avoid the necrotic groin tissue after vulvar cancer (Deppe et al. 1984; Hegarty et al. 1969). If this is not possible, the use of an autologous vascular graft is strongly preferred and coverage with vital tissue is very important.

With carotid artery rupture the situation is often dramatic, and in most cases the solution has been ligation of the artery. This can usually be done without sequelae, at least when the common carotid artery has ruptured (Ketcham and Hoye 1965; McCall et al. 1959), but obviously there is a risk of the development of stroke, even fatal (Dibbell and Gowen 1965; McCready et al. 1983). Wylie (1983) recommended ligation only in cases where the collateral situation was adequate, and otherwise reconstruction of the artery. The adequacy of the collaterals, however, is difficult to estimate (at least if there is a low stump pressure), and there are patients with such an extensive necrotic field that any type of reconstruction would be a high risk. Of 47 carotid ruptures reported in the literature, eight resulted in immediately fatal bleeding and 39 were ligated (Dibbell and Gowen 1965; Ketcham and Hoye 1965; Fajardo and Lee 1975; Marcial-Rojas and Castro 1962; McCall et al. 1959; McCready et al. 1983). Of the 39 patients in whom the artery was ligated, 29 had no sequelae (74%), six died (15%), and four developed a permanent neurologic deficit (10%).

Patients with radiated vessels and fibrotic periarterial tissue can be technically very difficult for the surgeon. This is the case, for instance, when dense fibrotic tissue has developed around the iliac vessels after pelvic radiation for gynecologic malignancy or around the subclavian artery after radiation for mammary carcinoma. In such cases, an extra-anatomic reconstructive solution of the problem is often recommendable, simplifying the situation for the surgeon and diminishing the risk of complications for the patient. There may also be poor graft inclusion in the radiated tissue with a risk of infection. In many cases, however, the stenotic or occlusive process is rather limited, and percutaneous transluminal angioplasty can be considered the method of choice; it has been used with success on both iliac and subclavian arteries (von Arlart and von Dewitz 1983; Bergqvist et al. 1987; Guthaner and Schmitz 1982; Saddekni et al. 1980).

References

Aarnoudse MW, Lamberts HB (1977) Arterial wall damage by X-rays and fast neutrons. Int J Radiat Biol 31:87–94

Amromin GD, Gildenhorn HL, Solomon RD, Nadkarni BB, Jacobs ML (1964) The synergism of X-irradiation and cholesterol-fat feeding on the development of coronary artery lesions. J Atheroscler Res 4:325–343

Annest LS, Anderson RP, Li W, Hafermann MD (1983) Coronary artery disease following mediastinal radiation therapy. J Thorac Cardiovasc Surg 85:253–257

Åstedt B, Bergentz S-E, Svanberg L (1974) Effect of irradiation on the plasminogen activator content in rat vessels. Experientia 30:1466–1467

Bansky G, Valli C, Häcki WH, Turina M (1984) Aorto-intestinale Fisteln. Bericht über vier Fälle. Schweiz Med Wochenschr 114:1263–1268

Benson EP (1973) Radiation injury to large arteries. Radiology 106:195–197

Bergqvist D (1987) Arterioenteric fistula. Review of vascular emergency. Acta Chir Scand 153:81–86

Bergqvist D, Forsberg L, Källerö S, Persson NH, Wikström I (1986) Radiation-induced carotid lesion caused transitory ischemic attacks (in Swedish). Läkartidingen 83:2943–2945

Bergqvist D, Jonsson K, Nilsson M, Takolander R (1987) Treatment of arterial lesions following radiation. Surg Gynecol Obstet 165:116–120

Borsanyi SJ (1962) Rupture of the carotids following radical neck surgery in radiated patients. Eye Ear Nose Throat Mon 41:531–533

Bosniak MA, Hardy MA, Quint J, Ghossein NA (1969) Demonstration of the effect of irradiation on canine bowel using in vivo photographic magnification angiography. Radiology 93:1361–1368

Budin JA, Casarella WJ, Harisladis L (1976) Subclavian artery occlusion following radiotherapy for carcinoma of the breast. Radiology 118:169–173

Butler MJ, Lane RHS, Webster JHH (1980) Irradiation injury to large arteries. Br J Surg 67:341–343

Cohn KE, Stewart JR, Fajardo LF, Hancock EW (1967) Heart disease following radiation. Medicine Baltimore 46:281–298

Colquhoun J (1966) Hypoplasia of the abdominal aorta following therapeutic irradiation in infancy. Radiology 86:454–456

Conley JJ (1953) The prevention of carotid artery hemorrhage by the use of rotating tissue flaps. Surgery 34:186–194

Conomy JP, Kellermeyer RW (1975) Delayed cerebrovascular consequences of therapeutic radiation. Cancer 36:1702–1708

Crummy AB, Hellman S, Stansel HC, Hukill PB (1965) Renal hypertension secondary to unilateral radiation damage relieved by nephrectomy. Radiology 84:108–111

Darmody WR, Thomas LM, Gurdjian ES (1967) Postirradiation vascular insufficiency syndrome. Neurology 17:1190–1192

Dencker H, H:son Holmdahl K, Lunderquist A, Olivecrona H, Tylén U (1972) Mesenteric angiography in patients with radiation injury of the bowel after pelvis irradiation. AJR 114:476–481

Deppe G, Malviya V, Smith P, Zbella E, Pildes R (1984) Limb salvage in recurrent vulvar carcinoma after rupture of the femoral artery. Gynecol Oncol 19:120–124

Dibbell DG, Gowen GF (1965) Observations on postoperative carotid hemorrhage. Am J Surg 109:765–770

Dollinger MR, Lavine DM, Foye LV (1966) Myocardial infarction due to postirradiation fibrosis of the coronary arteries. JAMA 195:176–179

Eisenberg RL, Hedgcock MW, Wara WM, Jeffrey RB (1978) Radiation-induced disease of the carotid artery. West J Med 129:500–503

Elerding SC, Fernandez RN, Grotta JC et al. (1981) Carotid artery disease following external cervical irradiation. Ann Surg 194:609–615

Estrada FP, Tachovsky TJ, Orr RM, Boylan JJ, Kram BW (1983) Primary aortoduodenal fistula following radiotherapy. Surg Gynecol Obstet 156:646–650

Fajardo LF, Lee A (1975) Rupture of major vessels after radiation. Cancer 36:904–913

Fehér J (1965) Myocardial infarction following radiation. Lancet 2:643–644

Fonkalsrud EW, Sanchez M, Zerubavel R, Mahoney A (1977) Serial changes in arterial structure following radiation therapy. Surg Gynecol Obstet 145:395–400

Fraumeni JF, Herweg JC, Kissane JM (1967) Panaortitis complicating Hodgkin's disease. Ann Intern Med 67:1242–1248

Georgelin M, Lichtenstein H, Singer B, Bodin F (1973) Hémorragie digestive massive par perforation ulcéreuse dans l'aorte abdominale. Nouv Presse Med 2:3046

Gerlock AJ, Goncharenko VA, Ekelund L (1977) Radiation-induced stenosis of the renal artery causing hypertension: case report. J Urol 118:1064–1065

Glick B (1972) Bilateral carotid occlusive disease following irradiation for carcinoma of the vocal cords. Arch Pathol 93:352–355

Glicksman AS, Nickson JJ (1973) Acute and late reactions to irradiation in the treatment of Hodgkin's disease. Arch Intern Med 131:369–373

Gold H (1961) Production of arteriosclerosis in the rat. Arch Pathol 71:268–273

Gross L, Manfredi OL, Frederick WC (1969) Radiation-induced major vascular occlusion in a patient cured of widespread metastases of nasopharyngeal origin. Radiology 93:664–666

Guthaner DF, Schmitz L (1982) Percutaneous transluminal angioplasty of radiation-induced arterial stenoses. Radiology 144:77–78

Hatcher PA, Thomson HJ, Ludgate SN, Small WP, Smith AN (1985) Surgical aspects of intestinal injury due to pelvic radiotherapy. Ann Surg 201:470–475

Hayward RH (1972) Arteriosclerosis induced by radiation. Surg Clin N Am 52:359–366

Hegarty JC, Linton PC, McSweeney ED (1969) Revascularization of the lower extremity through the obturator canal. Arch Surg 98:35–38

Heidenberg WJ, Lupovitch A, Tarr N (1966) "Pulseless disease" complicating Hodgkin's disease. A case apparently caused by radiotherapy. JAMA 195:194–197

Hopewell JW (1974) The late vascular effects of radiation. Br J Radiol 47:157–158

Hopewell JW (1980) The importance of vascular damage in the development of late radiation effects in normal tissues. In: Meyn R, Withers R (eds) Radiation biology in cancer research. Raven, New York, pp 449–459

Hopewell JW, Wright EA, Path FC (1970) The nature of latent cerebral irradiation damage and its modification by hypertension. Br J Radiol 43:161–167

Huff H, Sanders EM (1972) Coronary-artery occlusion after radiation. N Engl J Med 286:780

Hughes WF, Carson CL, Laffaye HA (1984) Subclavian artery occlusion 42 years after mastectomy and radiotherapy. Am J Surg 147:698–700

Iqbal SM, Hanson EL, Gensini GG (1977) Bypass graft for coronary arterial stenosis following radiation therapy. Chest 71:664–666

Johnson AG, Lane B, Harding Rains AJ, O'Connell D, Ramsay NW (1969) Large artery damage after X-radiation. Br J Radiol 42:937–939

Joseph DL, Shumrick DL (1973) Risks of head and neck surgery in previously irradiated patients. Arch Otolaryngol 97:381–384

Kagan AR, Bruce DW, Di Chiro G (1971) Fatal foam cell arteritis of the brain after irradiation for Hodgkin's disease: angiography and pathology. Stroke 2:232–238

Kaufman B, Lapham LW, Shealy CN, Pearson OH (1966) Transphenoidal yttrium-90 pituitary ablation. Radiation damage to the internal carotid arteries. Acta Radiol Ther Phys 5:17–25

Ketcham AS, Hoye RC (1965) Spontaneous carotid artery hemorrhage after head and neck surgery. Am J Surg 110:649–655

Kinsella TJ, Bloomer WD (1980) Tolerance of the intestine to radiation therapy. Surg Gynecol Obstet 151:273–284

Kirkpatrick JB (1967) Pathogenesis of foam cell lesions in irradiated arteries. Am J Pathol 50:291–300

Konings AWT, Hardonk MJ, Wieringa RA, Lamberts HB (1975) Initial events in radiation-induced atheromatosis. I. Activation of lysosomal enzymes. Strahlentherapie 150:444–448

Kretschmer G, Niederle B, Polterauer P, Waneck R (1986) Irradiation-induced changes in the subclavian and axillary arteries after radiotherapy for carcinoma of the breast. Surgery 99:658–663

Kwon T-H, Boronow RC, Swan RW, Hardy JD (1978) Arterio-enteric fistula following pelvic radiation: a case report. Gynecol Oncol 6:474–478

Lamberts HB, de Boer WGRM (1963) Contributions to the study of immediate and early X-ray reactions with regard to chemoprotection. VII. X-ray-induced atheromatous lesions in the arterial wall of hypercholesterolaemic rabbits. Int J Radiat Biol 6:343–350

Lee DH, Sapire D, Markowitz R, Gruskin A (1976) Radiation injury to abdominal aorta and iliac artery sustained in infancy. S Afr Med J 17:658–660

Levinson SA, Close MB, Ehrenfeld WK, Stoney J (1973) Carotid artery occlusive disease following external cervical irradiation. Arch Surg 107:395–397

Liegl O (1967) Über die Folgen einer Strahlenüberdosis am Hals. Ein Beitrag zum Syndrom des doppelseitigen Karotidenverschlusses. Z Kreislauf-Forsch 56:221–234

Liegl O (1975) Doppelseitiger Verschluß der großen Halsgefäße nach Röntgenbestrahlung in der Kindheit. Klin Monatsbl Augenheilkd 167:704–714

Lindsay S, Kohn HI, Dakin RL, Jew J (1962) Aortic arteriosclerosis in the dog after localized aortic X-irradiation. Circulation 10:51–60

Loeffler RK (1975) Subclavian artery occlusion following radiation therapy. A case history. Invest Radiol 10:391–393

Marcial-Rojas RA, Castro JR (1962) Irradiation injury to elastic arteries in the course of treatment in neoplastic disease. Ann Otol Rhinol Laryngol 71:945–958

Mavor GE, Kasenally AT, Harper DR, Woodruff PWH (1973) Thrombosis of the subclavian-axillary artery following radiotherapy for carcinoma of the breast. Br J Surg 60:983–985

McCall JW, Whitaker CW, Hendershot EL (1959) Rupture of the common carotid artery following radical neck surgery in radiated cases. Arch Otolaryngol 69:431–434

McConnel CS, Marlowe FI (1972) Postoperative perforation of the carotid artery by the hyoid bone. Arch Otolaryngol 95:282–283

McCready RA, Hyde GL, Bivins BA, Mattingly SS, Griffen WO (1983) Radiation-induced arterial injuries. Surgery 93:306–312

McEniery P, Dorosti K, Schiarone V, Pedrick T, Sheldon W (1987) Clinical and angiographic arteries of coronary artery disease after chest irradiation. Am J Cardiol 60:1020–1024

McGill CW, Holder TM, Smith TH, Ashcraft KW (1979) Postradiation renovascular hypertension. J Pediatr Surg 14:831–833

McReynolds RA, Gold GL, Roberts WC (1976) Coronary heart disease after mediastinal irradiation for Hodgkin's disease. Am J Med 60:39–45

Nardelli E, Fiaschi A, Ferrari G (1978) Delayed cerebrovascular consequences of radiation to the neck. Arch Neurol 35:538–540

Ormerod LP (1976) Acquired coarctation of the aorta – a long-term complication of irradiation. Br Med J 2:977

Painter MJ, Chutorian AM, Hilal SK (1975) Cerebrovasculopathy following irradiation in childhood. Neurology 25:189–194

Pepin B, Haguenau M, Goldstein B, Theron J, Bacourt F (1976) Deux cas de sténose post-radique des gros troncs artériels cérébraux. Ann Med Interne (Paris) 127:193–201

Poon TP, Kanshepolsky J, Tchertkoff V (1968) Rupture of the aorta due to radiation injury. JAMA 205:167–170

Poulias GE, Giannopoulos GD, Frangagis E (1967) Selective constriction of the profunda femoris as a postradiotherapy sequel. Report of a case. Radiology 89:127–128

Rasmussen S, Døssing M, Walbom-Jørgensen S (1978) Coronary heart disease – a possible risk in megavoltage therapy? Acta Med Scand 203:237–239

Reiter D, Piccone BR, Littman P, Lisker SA (1979) Tracheoinnominate artery fistula as a complication of radiation therapy. Otolaryngol Head Neck Surg 87:185–189

Rheudasil M, Chuang V, Amersen R (1988) Duodenocaval fistula: case report and literature review (1988). Ann Surg 54:169–171

Roscher AA, Steele BC, Woodard JS (1966) Carotid artery rupture after irradiation of larynx. Arch Otolaryngol 83:90–94

Rosenfeld JC, Savarese RP, De Laurentis DA (1987) Management of extremity ischemia secondary to radiation therapy. J Cardiovasc Surg 28:266–269

Ross HB, Sales JEL (1972) Post-irradiation femoral aneurysm treated by iliopopliteal bypass via the obturator foramen. Br J Surg 59:400–405

Rotman M, Seidenberg B, Rubin I, Botstein C, Bosniak M (1969) Aortic arch syndrome secondary to radiation in childhood. Arch Intern Med 124:87–90

Rubin E, Camara J, Grayzel DM, Zak FG (1963) Radiation-induced cardiac fibrosis. Am J Med 34:71–75

Saddekni S, Sniderman K, Hilton S, Sos T (1980) Percutaneous transluminal angioplasty of nonatherosclerotic lesions. AJR 135:975–982

Sams A (1965) Histological changes in the larger blood vessels of the hind limb of the mouse after X-irradiation. Int J Radiat Biol 9:165–174

Savlov ED, Nahhas WA, May AG (1969) Iliac and femoral arteriosclerosis following pelvic irradiation for carcinoma of the ovary. Obstet Gynecol 34:345–351

Servo A, Puranen M (1978) Moyamoya syndrome as a complication of radiation therapy. J Neurosurg 48:1026–1029

Sheehan JF (1944) Foam cell plaques in the intima of irradiated small arteries (one hundred to five hundred microns in external diameter). Arch Pathol 37:297–308

Silverberg GD, Britt RH, Goffinet DR (1978) Radiation-induced carotid artery disease. Cancer 41:130–137

Sinzinger H, Firbas W, Cromwell M (1983) Strahlenvaskulopathie – bedingt durch Änderung der gefäßeigenen Prostacyklinsynthese? Wien Klin Wochenschr 95:761–765

Staab GE, Tegtmeyer CJ, Constable WC (1976) Radiation-induced renovascular hypertension. AJR 126:634–637

St Louis EL, McLoughlin MJ, Wortzman G (1974) Chronic damage to medium and large arteries following irradiation. J Can Assoc Radiol 25:94–104

Thomas E, Forbus WD (1959) Irradiation injury to the aorta and the lung. Arch Pathol 67:256–263

Tracy GP, Brown DE, Johnson LW, Gottlieb AJ (1974) Radiation-induced coronary artery disease. JAMA 228:1660–1662

Vetto J, Culp S, Smythe T et al. (1987) Iliac arterial-enteric fistulas occurring after pelvic irradiation. Surgery 101:643–647

von Arlart IP, von Dewitz H (1983) Perkutane transluminale Angioplastik bei strahleninduzierter Beckenarterienstenose. Fortschr Rontgenstr 138:247–249

von Breit A (1969) Arteriographie vor und nach Tumorbestrahlung. Fortsch Rontgenstr 111:329–344

von Krückemeyer K (1973) Doppelseitiger Karotisverschluß nach Bestrahlung. Arztl Prax 27:1294

Wright TL, Bresnan MJ (1976) Radiation-induced cerebrovascular disease in children. Neurology 26:540–543

Wylie EJ (1983) Minisymposium: unusual problems in carotid surgery. Overview. Surgery 93:297–298

Vascular Injuries Due to Noninvasive Procedures

Types of Injury

Complications due to noninvasive procedures can be arterial occlusion induced by tourniquet, arterial occlusion induced by compression stockings, compartment syndrome because of the patient's position during surgery, or compartment syndrome after the use of pneumatic antishock trousers.

Mechanisms of Injury

In some arteriosclerotic patients, especially those with diabetes mellitus or Mönckeberg's medial calcinosis, it may be impossible to compress the arteries with a *tourniquet* or to induce a bloodless field with pressures of above 450 mm Hg (Jeyaseelan et al. 1981; Klenerman and Lewis 1976). This phenomenon is more common in the lower extremities and was seen in 10 out of 1500 patients undergoing ankle pressure measurement (Hobbs et al. 1974). It is therefore not astonishing that the pneumatic tourniquet may cause rupture of arteriosclerotic plaques in rare cases, thereby giving rise to the development of an occlusive thrombus (Giannestras et al. 1977; Irvine and Chan 1986; McAuley et al. 1984; Rush et al. 1987; Fig. 1). The cases hitherto published are summarized in Table 1.

Compression stockings are used to decrease edema formation in patients with swelling in the lower extremities for various reasons, as well as for prophylaxis against postoperative deep vein thrombosis. Although the pressure is low, the increased venous flow velocity produces a good thromboprophylactic effect, at least in low-risk surgery such as abdominal or gynecologic procedures. Two cases have been reported in which arterial thrombosis was most probably caused by graduated elastic compression stockings used for thromboprophylaxis (Heath et al. 1987). In both, however, there was a tourniquet effect of the stockings, in one because the stocking had been rolled to become a constricting band, in the other because of the development of considerable leg edema.

Dihydroergotamine, also used to increase venous flow velocity and therefore used thromboprophylactically, may in rare cases give rise to severe ischemia (for discussion see Lindblad 1988). This mechanism will not be further discussed here.

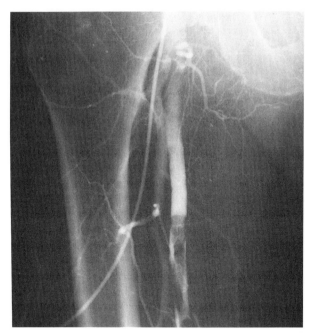

Fig. 1. Occlusion of the superficial femoral artery caused by a torniquet during bloodless field surgery

of compartment syndrome: diminished osteofascial volume, increased compartmental content for various reasons, and externally applied pressure (Table 2).

In this context, only the syndrome caused by compression during prolonged anesthesia in the knee-chest or lithotomy positions will be discussed. The pathophysiological background is the ischemic changes in muscles and nerves, which occur much more rapidly than in the skin. Irreversible changes are seen within 4–6 h. The ischemic changes within the muscles lead to increased microvascular permeability, which in turn leads to increased compartmental pressure exaggerating the ischemic injury to both muscles and nerves. The local end result may be Volkmann's contracture, known for more than 100 years (von Volkmann 1881). When the irreversible changes are extensive the prerequisite for a more generalized syndrome is filled, characterized by myoglobinuria, acute renal failure, metabolic acidosis, hyperkalemia, and shock. In recent years the syndrome has been called rhabdomyolysis (Gabow et al. 1982). Not only the extremity, but also the patient's life is threatened.

In 1953, Gordon and Newman described a 35-year-old male patient who developed a "lower nephron syndrome" after a prolonged period in the knee-chest position. The patient underwent a hemilaminectomy at the level of the fifth lumbar vertebra, and because of his obesity and height he was placed in the knee-chest position to obtain maximal widening of the intervertebral spaces. This position resulted in compression of the calf muscles from the patient's thighs and buttocks. Postoperatively, he developed swelling of the lower extremities and successively

Table 1. Patients with arterial lesions after the use of tourniquets for bloodless field reported in the literature

Author	Sex	Age (years)	Operation	Tourniquet Pressure (mm Hg)	Duration (min)	Time to diagnosis of ischemia	Diagnosis of ischemia	Operation	Outcome
Giannestras et al. (1977)	F	43	Correction of foot deformity bilaterally	500	70	Immediately	Clinical, doppler, angiography	TEA of plaque in a. femoralis superficialis + vein graft	Good
McAuley et al. (1984)	M	60	Total knee replacement, left	?	?	3–12 h	Clinical, angiography	Excision of segment of a. femoralis superficialis with intimal tear; end-to-end anastomosis	AK amp
Rush et al. (1987)	M	58	Total knee replacement, right	?	90	4 h	Clinical, angiography	Femoropopliteal vein bypass; fasciotomy	Good
Irvine and Chan (1986)	M	74	Tibial osteotomy	?	?	Immediately	Thrombectomy	Amputation	

Table 2. Causes of compartment syndrome

---

1. Diminished osteofascial volume
   a) Closure of fascial defects
   b) Excessive traction
   c) Burn injuries

2. Increased compartmental content
   a) Hemorrhage
   b) Increased capillary filtration
      – Increased capillary permeability
      – Increased capillary pressure
      – Diminished serum osmolarity
   c) Pressure infusion
   d) Muscular hypertrophy

3. Externally applied pressure
   a) Plaster of Paris
   b) Compression of extremities during anesthesia or drug abuse
   c) Pneumatic antishock garments

---

oliguria and anuria, and he died on the seventh postoperative day in renal failure. The authors concluded that it "appears most probable that the muscle damage from an unusual operative position was the basis for the development." Pressures of 105–240 mm Hg within the anterior tibial muscle during this position have been measured (Mubarak and Hargens 1981). Some cases have since been reported where the compartment syndrome occurred after operations in the lithotomy position; a summary is given in Table 3. The relatively young age of these patients is noteworthy and may indicate that an intact muscle mass is a prerequisite for the syndrome to develop.

In the lithotomy position there is a combination of pressure of the extremity against the leg brace, reducing the compartmental capacity, and elevation of the limb with reduced arterial perfusion. There may also be compression of the popliteal artery. During prolonged surgery other factors may coexist which increase the risk of a compartmental syndrome: hypothermia, hypovolemia with low flow because of fluid undersubstitution, local tissue injury, and pharmacologic vasoconstriction.

Since the beginning of the 1970s pneumatic antishock trousers have been used in the treatment of hemorrhagic shock as well as in the control of bleeding from pelvic fractures (Cutler and Daggett 1971; Flint et al. 1979). This form of treatment has been used frequently, and few complications associated with its use have been reported. Through the years there have been some case reports on the development of a severe compartment syndrome after release of the pressure in the garments. The cases are summarized in Table 4. The patients have all been young men, which reflects the trauma situation. The compartmental pressures were measured in all patients but one, often with very high values, or more than 100 mm Hg. The combination of the compartment syndrome with necrotic muscles and sepsis in some of the patients and the severe trauma probably contribute to the poor prognosis, with death having occurred in three of the seven patients. Two patients underwent amputation, one had a bilateral foot drop, and

Table 3. Reported cases of compartment syndrome in the legs after operation with patients in lithotomy position

Author	Sex	Age	Operation	Duration of procedure	Fasciotomy	Renal failure	Dialysis	Outcome
Goldberg et al. (1980)	M	52	Urethral stricture repair	6 h	b	+	+	Discharged with normal creatinine
Khalil (1987)	M	23	Total colectomy	7 h	+, bilateral ca. 12 h			3 months hyperesthesia
Leff and Shapiro (1979)	M	38	Urethroplasty (post-trauma)	6.5 h	+, bilateral ca. 24 h			Skin necrosis
Lydon and Spielman (1984)	F	44	Resection of pelvic tumor	9 h	+, bilateral several hours	+	+	Muscle weakness
Ready and Kaye (1984)	M [a]	65	Radical prostatectomy (cancer)	?	+, bilateral several hours			Drop foot
Sehlin et al. (1985)	M	20	Operation ad modum Soave (Hirschsprung's disease)	7 h	+, left side ca. 24 h			Skin transplantation
Bergqvist et al., unpublished	M	57	Bricker bladder (cancer)	8 h	+, bilateral, 21 h			Muscle fibrosis, left leg

[a] Patient had had a right-sided femoropopliteal bypass 6 years previously.
[b] Extreme tenderness, swelling, pain in both legs but no fasciotomy.

Table 4. Reported patients who developed compartment syndrome after pneumatic antishock garment application

Author	Sex	Age	Indications for garment	Pressure (mm Hg)	Duration of application	Fasciotomy	Renal failure	Dialysis	Outcome
Bass et al. (1983)	M	27	Stab wound	105	12 h	+, bilateral 24 h	+		Death, day 1
	M	25	Auto-pedestrian accident; unstable pelvis	105	24 h	+, right 24 h	+	+	Death, day 1
Brotman et al. (1982)	M	21	Automobile accident	10	ca. 4 h	+, left			Good
Godbout et al. (1984)	M	20	Automobile accident	90–35	ca. 4 h	+, bilateral a few hours	+		Death, day 7
Johnson (1981)	M	21	Motorcycle accident	?	3.5 h	+, bilateral	+	+	Resection of entire anterior compartments.
Maull et al. (1981)	M	26	Fall; unstable pelvis	105	48 h	+, left 24 h			AK amp
	M	45	Automobile accident; lower-extremity injury	15	28 h	+, bilateral; early			AK amp, right
Williams et al. (1982)	M	18	Knife laceration	?	ca. 2 h	+, bilateral			Bilateral foot drop

AK above knee.

only one recovered from the situation without sequelae. The compartment syndrome may be related to direct pressure on the tissues with decreased blood flow and to increased venous pressure. As the patients are traumatized and in hypotension, there are other risk factors for a decreased perfusion.

Incidence

The frequency of all the above-mentioned injuries is very low, only a few cases of each having been reported in the current literature.

Symptoms and Signs

Acute arterial occlusion after tourniquet and compression stockings does not differ from other types of arterial occlusions, and for a correct and fast diagnosis it is important to keep the possibility in mind.

The diagnosis of compartment syndrome is difficult. The clinical symptoms and signs are:
– Disproportionate pain, typical for all the patients described. In fact, there is no reason whatsoever why these patients should have pain in their legs. Complaints of pain should remind the surgeon of the possibility that a compartment syndrome is developing.
– Swelling and tenseness within a muscular compartment
– Weakness of muscles within the compartment, which, however, is a rather late sign (Hayden 1983)
– Severe muscle tenderness
– Accentuation of pain on passive stretching
– Hypoesthesia, paresthesia, and subsequent anesthesia. This sign between the first and second toe is an early manifestation of injury to the deep peroneal nerve. The first sensory losses are those of soft touch and proprioception.

One important fact is that peripheral pulses remain intact until the pressure within the compartment approaches blood pressure, which means that normal peripheral pulses by no means exclude the possibility of a compartment syndrome. In fact, although the pressure elevation is sufficient to occlude arterioles, it only rarely increases above the pressure in large arteries (Mubarak et al. 1978; Mubarak and Hargens 1983). Experimentally, direct measurements of microvascular blood pressures have shown that the blood pressure in 5–10μm vessels ranges between 20 and 30 mm Hg, and therefore compartmental pressures of more than 30 mm Hg will probably reduce microvascular blood flow (Akeson et al. 1981; Reneman et al. 1981). As a matter of fact, irreversible muscle damage occurs at compartmental pressures of 50–55 mm Hg for a duration of 4–8 h (Mubarak and Hargens 1983).

The *diagnosis* can in most cases be made on a clinical basis, and a high index of suspicion should lead to early treatment. If there are facilities to perform intracompartmental pressure measurements, these may be helpful but they should not delay treatment. If these are not routine measurements they may be more confusing than helpful. There are three principal ways of measuring compartmental pressure: with the help of a wick catheter, with the continuous infusion technique, or with a solid state transducer catheter (Matsen et al. 1981; McDermott et al. 1984; Mubarak and Hargens 1981). Normal pressure is low, and the normal value is itself a matter of discussion (Guyton et al. 1981; Wiederhielm 1981). There are some variations in the pressure limits for the diagnosis of a compartmental syndrome in the literature, but a pressure exceeding 30–40 mm Hg in combination with one or more of the symptoms and signs clearly indicates the need for fasciotomy. Increased body temperature usually indicates muscle necrosis.

There is no indication for angiography as a diagnostic tool for compartment syndrome. If angiography is done, there is a smooth tapering of the arteries, their diameter successively diminishing as the tissue pressure increases (Fig. 2). One differential diagnosis which may be very difficult is deep vein thrombophlebitis with the development of a phlegmasia alba dolens. If phlebography is done, the picture is rather typical, with nonfilling of the veins within the compartment and deviated flow through superficial veins.

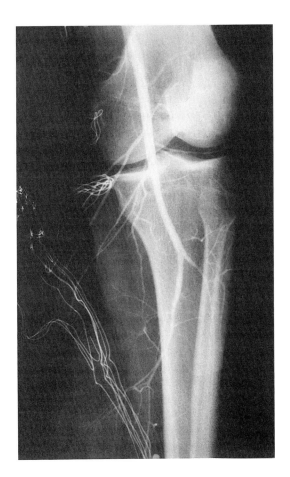

Fig. 2. The successive tapering of arteries in a lower limb with a compartment syndrome

Prevention

There is a risk of vascular occlusion when tourniquets are used to obtain a bloodless field in patients with arteriosclerotic vessels. It is important to be aware of the potential problem and to report cases of vascular injuries. Rush et al. (1987) recommend not using tourniquets in cases of knee surgery when there are no popliteal or distal pulses, or, if a tourniquet is used, they insist at least upon heparinizing the patient. So far, no firm recommendation can be made as to when to use and when not to use a tourniquet or as to whether heparinization is of any value. Calcifications seen on plain roentgenograms indicate medial calcinosis, and special care should be taken with such patients (Irvine and Chan 1986; Jeyaseelan et al. 1981; Savastano 1980). In all patients undergoing lower extremity surgery the preoperative history must also emphasize vascular problems (intermittent claudication, rest pain), and distal pulses must be palpated before and after the use of the tourniquet. If there is reason to suspect that the arterial circulation is impaired (history, decreased pulses, lowered ankle-brachial pressure indices) a vascular surgeon should be consulted before the orthopedic procedure is performed.

Compartment syndrome from compression during anesthesia can be avoided. Although the exact maximal safe time for legs in a lithotomy position is not known, a prolongation of the operation for more than 5–6 h should indicate complete release of all pressure and very careful postoperative observation of the patient; care must be taken not to compress the popliteal artery during the operation. In patients with some swelling and pain but with no neurologic symptoms we have seen prompt relief of symptoms after infusion of mannitol (200–400 ml, 30–60 g). Mannitol has two effects of possible benefit: it induces an osmotic diuresis and it acts as a superoxide radical scavenger (Buchbinder et al. 1981; Hutton et al. 1982; Shah et al. 1981). Through reduction of the free radicals muscle cell damage may be reduced.

When there is suspicion of compartment syndrome, compression bandages and elevation of the legs are contraindicated, as these maneuvers decrease the arterial perfusion pressure even more. If myoglobinuria is suspected, a high urinary output may decrease the nephrotoxic effect.

The indications for pneumatic antishock garments must be kept very strict. In cases of pelvic fracture a suit compartment pressure of 40–60 mm Hg seems to be sufficient, and where pressure has been kept within this range, compartment syndrome has never been reported (Bass et al. 1983). Only antishock trousers with pressure-monitoring possibilities should be used, to minimize the risk of overinflation. Pressures higher than 40 mm Hg should be applied only rarely and only during prehospital transport (Godbout et al. 1984). Also, pressures in the range of 40–60 mm Hg should never be applied for more than 24 h (Bass et al. 1983). Trousers should be inflated from the distal direction and deflation done in the opposite direction. Patients with more than 2 h of high pressure inflation must be carefully observed. Abdominal compartment pressure must not exceed leg compartment pressure.

Treatment

In cases of arterial thrombosis due to tourniquet or other types of compression, the treatment is directed at proper reconstruction.

In cases of compartment syndrome the treatment is fasciotomy. There are several methods of performing this. It is necessary to adequately open all four compartments, and there is no reason not to open the skin as well. The skin incisions are easily closed later on, with or without a skin graft. When the fasciotomy is done it is also important to remove necrotic tissue and later in the course to make adequate revisions.

Rhabdomyolysis, myoglobinuria, and renal failure require intensive nephrologic treatment, which, however, falls outside the scope of this discussion. Temporary dialysis may be necessary as well.

References

Akeson W, Hargens A, Garfin S, Mubarak S (1981) Muscle compartment syndrome and snake bites. In: Hargens A (ed) Tissue fluid pressure and composition. Williams and Wilkins, Baltimore

Bass RR, Allison EJ, Reines HD, Yeager JC, Pryor WH (1983) Thigh compartment syndrome without lower-extremity trauma following application of pneumatic antishock trousers. Ann Emerg Med 12:382

Brotman S, Browner BD, Cox EF (1982) MAS trousers improperly applied causing a compartment syndrome in lower-extremity trauma. J Trauma 22:598–599

Buchbinder D, Karmody A, Leather R, Shah DM (1981) Hypertonic manitol. Arch Surg 116:414–421

Cutler BS, Daggett WM (1971) Application of the "G-suit" to the control of hemorrhage in massive trauma. Ann Surg 173:511–514

Flint LM, Brown A, Richardson JD et al. (1979) Definitive control of bleeding from severe pelvic fractures. Ann Surg 198:709–716

Gabow PA, Kachny WD, Kelleher SP (1982) The spectrum of rhabdomyolysis. Medicine (Baltimore) 61:141–152

Giannestras NJ, Cranley JJ, Lentz M (1977) Occlusion of the tibial artery after a foot operation. J Bone Joint Surg [Am] 59-A:682–683

Godbout B, Burchard KW, Slotman GJ, Gann DS (1984) Crush syndrome with death following pneumatic antishock garment application. J Trauma 24:1052–1056

Goldberg M, Stecker JF, Scarff JE, Wombolt DG (1980) Rhabdomyolysis associated with urethral stricture repair: report of a case. J Urol 124:730–731

Gordon BS, Newman W (1953) Lower nephron syndrome following prolonged knee-chest position. J Bone Joint Surg [Am] 35-A:674–768

Guyton A, Barber B, Moffatt D (1981) Theory of interstitial pressures. In: Hargens A (ed) Tissue fluid pressure and compositon. Williams and Wilkins, Baltimore, pp 11–19

Hayden JW (1983) Compartment syndromes. Early recognition and treatment. Postgrad Med 74:191–202

Heath D, Kents S, Johns D, Young T (1987) Arterial thrombosis associated with graduated-pressure antiembolic stockings. Br Med J 2:580

Hobbs JT, Yao ST, Lewis JD, Needham TN (1974) A limitation of the Doppler ultrasound method of measuring ankle systolic pressure. Vasa 3:160–162

Hutton M, Rhodes RS, Chapman G (1982) The lowering of postischemic compartment pressures with mannitol. J Surg Res 32:239–242

Irvine GB, Chan RNW (1986) Arterial calcification and tourniquets. Lancet 2:1217

Jeyaseelan S, Stevenson TM, Pfitzner J (1981) Tourniquet failure and arterial calcification. Anaesthesia 36:48–50

Johnson BE (1981) Anterior tibial compartment syndrome following use of MAST suit. Ann Emerg Med 10:209–210

Khalil IM (1987) Bilateral compartmental syndrome after prolonged surgery in the lithotomy position. J Vasc Surg 5:879–881

Klenerman L, Lewis JD (1976) Incompressible vessels. Lancet 1:811–812

Leff RG, Shapiro SR (1979) Lower-extremity complications of the lithotomy position: prevention and management. J Urol 122:138–139

Lindblad B (1988) Prophylaxis of postoperative thromboembolism with low dose heparin alone or in combination with dihydroergotamine. A review. Acta Chir Scand [Suppl] 543:31–42

Lydon JC, Spielman FJ (1984) Bilateral compartment syndrome following prolonged surgery in the lithotomy position. Anesthesiology 60:236–238

Maull KI, Capehart JE, Cardea JA, Haynes BW (1981) Limb loss following military anti-shock trousers (MAST) application. J Trauma 21:60–62

McAuley CE, Steed DL, Webster MW (1984) Arterial complications of total knee replacement. Arch Surg 119:960–962

Matsen F, Wyss C, King R (1981) The continuous infusion technique in the assessment of clinical compartment syndromes. In: Hargens A (ed) Tissue fluid pressure and composition. Williams and Wilkins, Baltimore, pp 255–259

McDermott AGP, Marble AE, Yabsley RH (1984) Monitoring acute compartment pressures with the STIC catheter. Clin Orthop 190:192–198

Mubarak S, Hargens A (1981) Clinical use of the Wick-catheter technique. In: Hargens A (ed) Tissue fluid pressure and composition. Williams and Wilkins, Baltimore, pp 261–268

Mubarak SJ, Hargens AL (1983) Acute compartment syndromes. Surg Clin North Am 63:539–565

Mubarak S, Owen CA, Hargens A, Garetto LP, Akeson HW (1978) Acute compartment syndromes; diagnosis and treatment with the use of the Wick catheter. J Bone Joint Surg [Am] 60-A:1091–1095

Reddy PK, Kaye KW (1984) Deep posterior compartmental syndrome: a serious complication of the lithotomy position. J Urol 132:144–145

Reneman R, Slaaf D, Lindbom L, Tangelder GJ, Arfors K-E (1981) Muscle blood-flow disturbances in compartment syndromes and the role of elevated total muscle-tissue pressure in these disturbances. In: Hargens A (ed) Tissue fluid pressure and composition. Williams and Wilkins, Baltimore, pp 209–214

Rush JH, Vidovich JD, Johnson MA (1987) Arterial complications of total knee replacement. The Australian experience. J Bone Joint Surg [Br] 69-B:400–402

Savastano AA (1980) Preoperative and postoperative considerations in knee joint replacement surgery. Appleton-Century-Crofts, New York, pp 41–47

Sehlin J, Dolk A, Holmström B, Netz P (1985) Patient developed compartment syndrome after Mb Hirschsprung operation (in Swedish). Lakartidningen 82:4323–4324

Shah DW, Powers SR, Stratton HH, Newell JC (1981) Effect of hypertonic mannitol on oxygen utilization in canine hind limbs following shock. J Surg Res 30:593–601

von Volkmann R (1881) Die ischaemischen Muskellähmungen und Kontrakturen. Zentralbl Chir 8:8091

Wiederhielm C (1981) The tissue pressure controversy: a semantic dilemma. In: Hargens A (ed) Tissue fluid pressure and composition. Williams and Wilkins, Baltimore, pp 11–19

Williams TM, Knopp R, Ellyson JH (1982) Compartment syndrome after anti-shock trouser use without lower-extremity trauma. J Trauma 22:595–597

Vascular Injuries in Orthopedic Surgery

Types of Injury

Acute injuries may be laceration, arterial occlusion, or microembolization. *Delayed injuries* may appear as pseudoaneurysms, arteriovenous fistulas, or foreign bodies in the vessel.

Causes of Injury

Laceration causing hemorrhage may occur during dissection close to the great vessels. Such injuries, occurring acutely and requiring urgent handling, are probably underreported when they are dealt with in an adequate way, leaving no or only minor sequelae. Arthroscopic meniscectomy may be complicated by laceration of the popliteal artery with severe hemorrhage (Jeffries et al. 1987). A more delayed type of injury causing hemorrhage can be instituted by pins, nails, and screws, with gradual erosion of the vessels. Buri (1971) reported on a young girl who died of bleeding, when a Kirschner pin through the sternoclavicular joint penetrated the intrapericardial part of the aorta, causing a cardiac tamponade. In a male patient, a Steinmann pin was used because of nonunion of a supracondylar femoral fracture, and after 9 days, bleeding occurred from erosion of the superficial femoral artery (Stein 1956). Similar delayed bleeding occurred in a patient with throchanteric reticulum cell sarcoma with a fracture, leading to hip disarticulation and double ligation of the femoral artery. Bleeding occurred 14 days postoperatively because of a hole in the femoral artery, relieved by ligation of the common iliac artery (Stein 1956). It cannot be excluded that infection plays an important role in the development of delayed hemorrhage, especially when there is erosion or necrosis of the vessels. Delayed bleeding within a week or two after arterial reconstructive surgery is almost exclusively caused by infection (Bergqvist and Källerö 1985; Bergqvist and Ljungström 1987).

Arterial occlusion may be caused by various factors. There may be damage to the arterial wall during the dissection procedure or from the use of retractors, especially when the operation is performed in a bloodless field. Operations in the knee region are potentially dangerous because of the very poor collateral circulation around the knee joint should the popliteal artery be occluded (Fig. 1). Injuries have been reported during knee arthroplasty (McAuley et al. 1984; Robson et al. 1975; Rush et al. 1987), but also after open meniscectomy (Ross 1951) as well as after arthroscopic meniscectomy (Jeffries et al. 1987). However, arthroscopic surgery is very rarely the cause of vascular lesions (Jackson 1983). On the other hand, if care is not taken, extravasation during arthroscopy may give rise to intrafascial

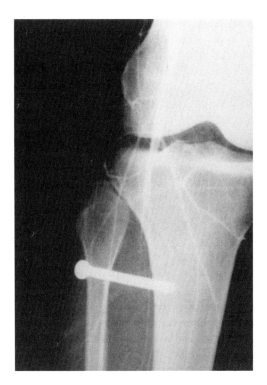

Fig. 1. The tibio-fibular joint of a 24-year-old woman, operated on for instability. Postoperatively she had extensive pain, and the foot showed no pulse, was cold, and had impaired mobility. Although the clinical picture was highly suggestive of ischemia, angiography and operation were delayed and blood flow was not restored until after 7 h. She developed sequelae in the form of muscle contractures

deposits, resulting in a compartment syndrome (Fruensgaard and Holm 1988; Nillius and Rooser 1983; Peek and Haynes 1984).

Another possible mechanism for arterial occlusion is external arterial compression from firm callus and/or scar tissue after corrective femoral osteotomies (Brown et al. 1968; Knight et al. 1980) or from fascial or scary structures after total knee replacement (Fortune 1986; Robson et al. 1975), especially if there is a tendency to overextension of the knee joint. Another causative factor is a cerclage including the artery.

McAuley et al. (1984) described the development of chronic ischemia in a patient who had undergone a total knee replacement 16 months previously. At angiography, a stenosis was found 1 cm proximal to the prosthesis. The patient later underwent reconstruction with a femorotibial reversed saphenous vein bypass. However, the cause relationship in this case is very difficult to establish. The patient was at the typical arteriosclerosis age (62 years) and the rapidity of the disease progress is of little value in solving the problem. In certain cases it cannot be excluded that an arteriosclerotic process may be accelerated or even induced by an operative trauma, but the evidence for a causal relationship is weak, and in fact weaker, the longer the interval between surgery and symptoms of impaired circulation. Under certain circumstances there may be stronger evidence for a cause relationship, when the condition occurs:

1. In young patients who have an otherwise healthy arterial system, including the contralateral side
2. In patients with no risk factors for arteriosclerosis

Microembolization: a nonocclusive thrombus, in itself not giving rise to ischemia, is a potential source of the process of microembolization. Microemboli may also arise from the thrombus inside a pseudoaneurysm (Falconer and Adar 1984).

Pseudoaneurysms may be the result of all sorts of arterial damage, leading to a self-limiting hemorrhage because of the tissue counterpressure. This condition has been described in the inferior lateral genicular artery after lateral meniscectomy (Fairbank and Jamieson 1951; Hooper and Spring 1953) and knee arthroplasty (Coventry et al. 1973); in the popliteal artery after both lateral and medial meniscectomies, also arthroscopic, and knee arthroplasty (Beck et al. 1986; Patrick 1963; Rush et al. 1987); in the deep femoral artery after intramedullary nailing of femoral fracture (Dickson 1968); in the superficial femoral artery after supracondylar osteotomy (Falconer and Adar 1984); in lumbar arteries after spinal fusion (Horton 1972); in posterior tibial arteries after foot stabilization procedures (Morris and Morse 1966; Webb-Jones 1955); in the peroneal artery after extirpation of a Brodie's abscess (Scott 1955) or fixation of a fracture with a tibial plate (Onursal et al. 1987); and in the ulnar artery after joint exploration (Thio 1972). Migration of a Kirschner wire used to stabilize a humeral fracture was the cause of an axillary artery pseudoaneurysm in one patient, described by Onursal et al. (1987).

Arteriovenous fistulae may also be seen after various types of orthopedic surgical procedures, the most dramatic, perhaps, developing after lumbar disk surgery (see p. 108). Other operations reported to have resulted in arteriovenous communications are correction of club foot deformity (Coughlin 1951; Webb-Jones 1955; Glasser and Bray 1949; Horton 1972), meniscectomy or knee arthroplasty (Crowley and Masterson 1984; Patrick 1963; Pritchard et al. 1977; Rush et al. 1987; Schlosser et al. 1982), leg amputation (Mason et al. 1936; Naylor 1950; Stuart 1929), hip adductor tenotomy (Griffiths 1955), foot arthrodesis (Higgs 1931; Ogilvie 1931), stabilization of foot fracture with Steinmann pin and stretch (Gamm 1942), and placement of an intramedullary femoral rod (between the superior gluteal vessels) (Creech et al. 1965).

Migration to vessels of orthopedic devices, thereby becoming foreign body emboli, is extremely rare, although the cardiovascular migration of foreign bodies in itself is a well-known phenomenon (Schechter and Gilbert 1969; Moncada et al. 1978). Nordback and Markkula (1985) described a 22-year-old male patient with multiple trauma in whom a clavicular fracture was treated with two Kirschner pins. At radiographic control one pin was located in the mediastinum, in what was thought to be the caval vein. At thoracotomy it was found to be placed inside the aorta, however, and it was extracted by being pushed through the aortic wall. It is also possible that the foreign body only penetrates the vessel wall without migrating totally into it. One patient died from perforation of the pulmonary artery by a Kirschner wire used to stabilize a sternoclavicular joint (Leonard and Gifford 1965). Pate and Wilhite (1969) described a male patient in whom a Kirschner wire migrated from the sternoclavicular joint to the pulmonary artery and to the outflow tract of the right ventricle. The wire was extracted and the postoperative course uneventful. Onursal et al. (1987) also described a case of a Kirschner wire that migrated to the pulmonary artery and was successfully extirpated. In one patient with roentgenologic evidence of medial migration of a Hagie pin used to stabilize the acromioclavicular joint, extirpation provoked severe hemorrhage, which at exploration was shown to emanate from the perforated subclavian artery (Sethi and Scott 1976).

Incidence

The incidence of vascular injuries during and after orthopedic surgical procedures is obviously low, but the true frequency is largely unknown and can probably be established only in a careful prospective study. In relation to the vast number of orthopedic operations performed, however, such injuries are not common. During the early 1950s there were no arterial injuries among 450 knee arthroplasties performed at the Mayo Clinic (Bryan et al. 1973), among 89 performed in Winnipeg (Gunston and MacKenzie 1976), and among 7073 performed in Syndey (quoted by Rush et al. 1987). To indicate the extent of the problem, only around 20 injuries during knee replacement are known from the literature. In the United States 45 000 knee arthroplasties are performed every year (McAuley et al. 1984).

Between 1970 and 1980, Schlosser et al. (1982) in Freiburg, West Germany, performed 3640 arterial reconstructions. Among these, 17 were due to iatrogenic complications after orthopedic surgery (total hip replacement in 12, spinal disk surgery in two, meniscectomy in three). The number has recently increased to 43 patients, so far presented in an abstract (Schlosser et al. 1987). Eighteen were seen after total hip replacement, eight after knee joint surgery, two after lumbar disk surgery, and 15 after fracture fixation. During the 30-year period 1955–1984 there were a total of 131 vascular injuries in the city of Malmö, Sweden (ca. 240 000 inhabitants). Seventy-one were iatrogenic but only four occurred during orthopedic surgery, all in the last 10-year period. Three occurred in the external iliac artery during hip reoperative procedures in patients who had previously undergone arthroplasty. In one patient the axillary artery was lacerated with a forceps during operation for an old humeral osteomyelitis (Bergqvist et al. 1987).

Hohf (1963) sent a questionnaire to 3500 members of the American Academy of Orthopedic Surgeons; 1163 replied. Two hundred and ninety of the responders had personal knowledge of a total of 352 arterial injuries. The most common type of arterial injury was laceration (249), followed by division (85) and obstruction (18). In 33 cases there were late complications in the form of arteriovenous fistulae (21) and pseudoaneurysms (12). The highest number of patients incurred their injuries during operations on the lumbar spine and the pelvis, this group also containing the highest number of untreated or unrecognized cases, reflected by a death rate of 23% (17/74). Injuries of the popliteal artery at the knee level, especially after meniscectomy, resulted in the highest frequency of major amputations (34%).

In Paris, Huard (1974) questioned 166 French orthopedic surgeons and received reports on 79 lesions, the lower extremity dominating with 63 cases (11 in hip and pelvis, 26 at the thigh level, and 26 below the knee).

Rush et al. (1987) sent a questionnaire about major vascular complications after total knee replacement during a 10-year period to 470 fellows of the Australian Orthopaedic Association. Among the 100 replies 12 cases were reported. Three of these were direct laceration of the popliteal artery, seven were femoral/popliteal artery thrombosis, and one each arteriovenous fistula (lateral geniculate vessels) and pseudoaneurysm. Of the five with direct trauma (laceration, pseudoaneurysm, and arteriovenous fistulae) vascular repair led to limb survival in all. Of the seven with thrombosis, one patient died, five ended up with amputations, and in one the outcome was unknown. Injuries to the popliteal artery are especially dangerous, and a delayed diagnosis can lead to loss of the limb.

A national survey of the complications to arthroscopy and arthroscopic surgery by the Arthroscopy Association of North America recorded six penetrating injuries to the popliteal artery in 118 590 reported arthroscopic procedures. Four of the six ended with amputation. Arden (1974) reported one patient with foot ischemia after performing 209 total knee replacements in 160 patients. The case was not specified. Coventry et al. (1973) had one patient with a pseudoaneurysm of the descending genicular artery among 261 patients with 317 geometric knee prostheses.

Prevention

As always, an adequate knowledge of topographic anatomy is of utmost importance in avoiding complications. But it is also important to remember the distorted anatomy that is at hand in cases of redo procedures. Harty and Kostowiecki (1965) have summarized the normal anatomy as well as various types of variations of the deep femoral and inferior lateral geniculate arteries, with special emphasis on what may happen during orthopedic operations. They also state an axiom that one should consider when performing bone screwing. There "should be maximal engagement but minimal protrusion." At primary operations most vessels are relatively mobile, except for the superficial femoral artery, which is fixed in its passage through the adductor canal. During surgery in this region special care must be taken. On insertion of various nails, screws, pins, tenotomy or chisel-type meniscectomy knives, and so on, due regard to the vessel anatomy is a must. With the arthoscopic removal of cartilage the risk for vessel injury should be minimal.

When using plaster of Paris, for instance after a corrective osteotomy, it is important to remove the plaster if there is any suspicion of ischemia whatsoever. In stabilizing operations on the foot, full exposure of the joint surfaces is safer than blind cutting. When foreign material is used it should be secured during its insertion to prevent migration, e.g., bending of Kirschner pins.

When operations have been performed near arteries or when a tourniquet has been used it is important to evaluate the vascular status postoperatively by inspection, palpation of pulses, and perhaps distal pressure measurement. Such a routine is recommended to ascertain that the circulatory status is unaltered compared with preoperatively, thereby excluding a major vascular injury during the surgical procedure. A single investigation is no guarantee, however, as thrombotic occlusion may take some time to develop. Early diagnosis and prompt treatment are important to improve the prognosis. The diagnosis of arterial spasm must never be made until a morphological lesion has been excluded.

Treatment

The aim is always to restore anatomy, and thereby function. The importance of restoring popliteal artery continuity is reflected in the high frequency of amputations seen when no treatment or late treatment is instituted (Rush et al. 1987; Patrick 1963). This is well known also from noniatrogenic injuries to the popliteal artery (Bergqvist et al. 1987; Bishara et al. 1986; Fabian et al. 1982; Jagges et al. 1982; Lim et al. 1980). In cases where there is a delay or where other priorities are present, an indwelling temporary shunt is recommended. When a shunt is used it is probably of value to heparinize the patient.

In unclear cases a rapid angiography is of value, but it is the responsibility of the surgeon to keep the delay until surgery to a minimum. The possibility of performing the angiographic examination on the operating table should be kept in mind.

In patients in whom foreign bodies have intruded into the arteries the percutaneous route can be used successfully for extirpation on many occasions.

References

Arden GP (1974) Complications of total knee replacement and their treatment. Excerpta Med Int Congr Ser 324:221–227

Beck DE, Robison JG, Hallett JW (1984) Popliteal artery pseudoaneurysm following arthroscopy. J Trauma 26:87–89

Bergqvist D, Källerö S (1985) Reoperation for postoperative haemorrhagic complications. Analysis of a 10-year series. Acta Chir Scand 151:17–22

Bergqvist D, Ljungström KG (1987) Haemorrhagic complications leading to reoperation after peripheral vascular surgery. A 14-year material. J Vasc Surg 6:134–139

Bergqvist D, Helfer M, Jensen N, Tägil M (1987) Trends in civilian vascular trauma during 30 years – a Swedish perspective. Acta Chir Scand 153:417–422

Bishara RA, Pasch AR, Lim LT et al. (1986) Improved results in the treatment of civilian vascular injuries associated with fractures and dislocations. J Vasc Surg 3:707–711

Brown R, Gore D, Sauter KE, Mueller KH (1986) Arterial obstruction of the femoral artery secondary to femoral osteotomy. J Bone Joint Surg 50-A:1444–1446

Bryan R, Peterson L, Combs J (1973) Polycentric knee arthroplasty. A preliminary report of postoperative complications in 450 knees. Clin Orthop 94:148–152

Buri P (1971) Iatrogene Schädigung von Blutgefäßen. Helv Chir Acta 38:151–155

Coughlin JJ (1951) Arterio-venous aneurysm of the foot following plantar fasciotomy. Northwest Med 50:772–773

Coventry MB, Upshaw JE, Riley LH, Finerman GAM, Turner RH (1973) Geometric total knee arthroplasty. Clin Orthop 94:117–184

Creech O, Gantt J, Wren H (1965) Traumatic arteriovenous fistula at unusual sites. Ann Surg 161:908–920

Crowley JG, Masterson R (1984) Popliteal arteriovenous fistula following meniscectomy. J Trauma 24:164–165

Dickson JW (1968) False aneurysm after intramedullary nailing of the femur. J Bone Joint Surg [Br] 50-B:144–145

Fabian TC, Turkleson ML, Connelly TL, Stone HH (1982) Injury to the popliteal artery. Am J Surg 143:225–228

Fairbank TJ, Jamieson ES (1951) A complication of lateral meniscectomy. J Bone Joint Surg [Br] 33-B:567–570

Falconer DP, Adar U (1984) Pseudoaneurysm secondary to a protruding screw as a result of normal growth and remodeling following supracondylar osteotomy. J Bone Joint Surg [Am] 60-A:1126–1128

Fortune W (1986) Complications of total and partial arthroplasty in the knee. In: Epps C (ed) Complications in orthopedic surgery. Lippincott, Philadelphia

Fruensgaard S, Holm A (1988) Compartment syndrome complicating arthroscopic surgery: brief report. J Bone Joint Surg 70B:146–147

Gamm KE (1942) Arteriovenous fistula. JAMA 119:134–135

Glasser ST, Bray HP (1949) Arteriovenous fistula. A case report emphasizing etiology. Industrial Med Surg 18:329–331

Griffiths DL (1955) Arterial injuries and orthopaedic operations. J Bone Joint Surg [Br] 37-B:369–370

Gunston FH, MacKenzie RI (1976) Complications of polycentric knee arthroplasty. Clin Orthop 120:11–17

Harty M, Kostowiecki M (1965) Vascular injuries in limb surgery. Surg Gynecol Obstet 121:339–342

Higgs SL (1931) Arterio-venous aneurysm of the posterior tibial vessels following operation for stabilizing the foot. Proc R Soc Med 24:1378–1379

Hohf RP (1963) Arterial injuries occurring during orthopaedic operations. Clin Orthop 28:21–37

Hooper RS, Spring WE (1953) Popliteal aneurysm after lateral meniscectomy. J Bone Joint Surg [Br] 35-B:272–274

Horton RE (1972) Arterial injuries complicating orthopaedic surgery. J Bone Joint Surg [Br] 54-B:323–327

Huard C (1974) Lésions vasculaires iatrogènes du membre inférieur. Rev Chir Orthop 60:[Suppl]36–40

Jackson RW (1983) Current concepts review. Arthroscopic surgery. J Bone Joint Surg [Am] 65-A:416–420

Jagges RC, Feliciano DV, Mattox KL, Graham JM, DeBakey ME (1982) Injury to popliteal vessels. Arch Surg 117:657–661

Jeffries JT, Gainor BJ, Allen WC, Cikrit D (1987) Injury to the popliteal artery as a complication of arthroscopic surgery. J Bone Joint Surg [Am] 69-A:783–785

Knight JL, Ratcliffe SS, Weber JK, Hansen ST (1980) Corrective osteotomy of femoral shaft malunion causing complete occlusion of the superficial femoral artery. A case report. J Bone Joint Surg [Am] 62-A:303–306

Leonard JW, Gifford RW (1965) Migration of a Kirschner wire from the clavicle into the pulmonary artery. Am J Cardiol 16:598–600

Lim LT, Michuda MMS, Flanigan DP, Pankovich A (1980) Popliteal artery trauma. Arch Surg 115:1021–1024

Mason JM, Pool RM, Collier JP (1936) The treatment of traumatic arteriovenous aneurysms. South Med J 29:248–257

McAuley CE, Steed DL, Webster MW (1984) Arterial complications of total knee replacement. Arch Surg 119:960–962

Moncada R, Matuga T, Unger E, Freeark R, Pizarro A (1978) Migratory traumatic cardiovascular foreign bodies. Circulation 57:186–189

Morris E, Morse TS (1966) Aneurysm of the posterior tibial artery after a foot stabilization procedure. J Bone Joint Surg [Am] 48-A:337–338

Naylor A (1950) Arteriovenous fistula complicating an amputation stump. Br Med J 2:928

Nillius A, Rooser B (1983) Acute compartment syndrome during knee arthroscopy (in Swedish). Lakartidningen 80:590

Nordback I, Markkula H (1985) Migration of Kirschner pin from clavicle into ascending aorta. Acta Chir Scand 151:177–179

Ogilvie WH (1931) Discussion of Higgs SL. Arterio-venous aneurysm of posterior tibial vessels following operation for stabilizing the foot. Proc R Soc Med 24:1378

Onursal E, Bedirhem A, Sonmez B, Kargi A, Barlas C (1987) Arterial complications following orthopaedic reconstructions. J Cardiovasc Surg (Torino) 28:731–733

Pate JW, Wilhite JL (1969) Migration of a foreign body from the sternoclavicular joint to the heart: a case report. Am Surg 35:448–449

Patrick J (1963) Aneurysm of the popliteal vessels after meniscectomy. J Bone Joint Surg [Br] 45-B:570–571

Peek R, Haynes D (1984) Compartment syndrome as a complication of arhtroscopy. A case report and a study of interstitial pressures. Am J Sports Med 12:464–468

Pritchard DA, Maloney JD, Barnhorst DA, Spittell JA (1977) Traumatic popliteal arterio-venous fistula. Arch Surg 112:849–852

Robson LJ, Walls CE, Swanson AB (1975) Popliteal artery obstruction following Shiers total knee replacement. Clin Orthop 109:130–133

Ross WT (1951) Injury to the popliteal artery during meniscectomy. J Bone Joint Surg [Br] 33-B:571

Rush JH, Vidovich JD, Johnson MA (1987) Arterial complications of total knee replacement. The Australian experience. J Bone Joint Surg [Br] 69-B:400–402

Schechter DC, Gilbert L (1969) Injuries of the heart and great vessels due to pins and needles. Thorax 24:246–253

Schlosser V, Spillner G, Breymann T, Urbanyi B (1982) Vascular injuries in orthopaedic surgery. J Cardiovasc Surg (Torino) 23:32–37

Schlosser V, Kuttler H, Kameda T (1987) Arterial injury during orthopedic and traumatological surgery. J Cardiovasc Surg (Torino) 28:46

Scott JH (1955) Traumatic aneurysm of the peroneal artery. J Bone Joint Surg [Br] 37-B:438–439

Sethi GK, Scott SM (1976) Subclavian artery laceration due to migration of a Hagie pin. Surgery 80:644–646

Stein AH (1956) Arterial injury in orthopaedic surgery. J Bone Joint Surg [Am] 38-A:669–676

Stuart DW (1929) Arterio-venous aneurysm following amputation. Br Med J 2:346

Thio RT (1972) False aneurysm of the ulnar artery after surgery employing a tourniquet. Am J Surg 123:604–605

Webb-Jones A (1955) Aneurysm after foot stabilization. J Bone Joint Surg [Br] 37-B:440–442

Hip Surgery and Vascular Trauma

Types of Injury

Vascular injury related to hip surgery may be acute, e.g., arterial or venous laceration, thrombotic stenosis-occlusion, or ischemia from division of collateral vessels, or it may be late developing, e.g., an arteriovenous fistula or a pseudoaneurysm.

Mechanisms of Injury

Several mechanisms of injury have been described, the main ones being as follows:
1. Laceration giving rise to hemorrhage, pseudoaneurysm (Figs. 1–3), or arteriovenous fistula may be due to:
   a) Direct injury from compression by a Hohmann retractor (Aust et al. 1981; Kroese and Møllerud 1975; Øvrum and Dahl 1979) or pin retractors (Lozman and Robbins 1983; Nachbur et al. 1979), drilling, a measuring stick

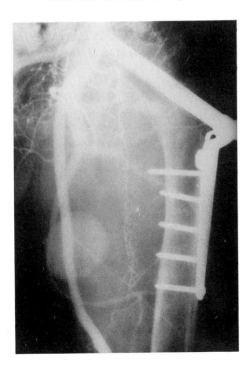

Fig. 1. Pseudoaneurysm detected around 8 months after treatment for intertrochanter fracture. Postoperatively the patient had a large hematoma and swelling of the leg. A bruit was heard, angiography giving the diagnosis. The deep femoral artery was ligated

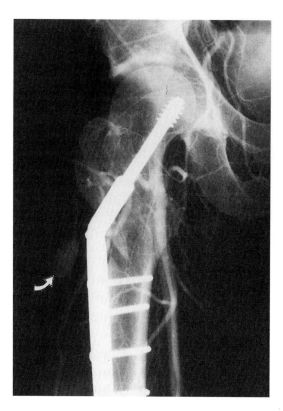

Fig. 2. Pseudoaneurysm (*arrow*) of the circumflex femoral artery developing some weeks after osteosynthesis for an intertrochanter fracture. The patient was treated with ligation

or reamer (Bergqvist et al. 1972; Mackenzie et al. 1983; von Eggert and Huland 1974), sharp spiculae formed by the cement (Aust et al. 1981; Bergqvist 1983; Dorr et al. 1974; Eriksson et al. 1971; Hopkins et al. 1983; Neumann and Berge 1985; Nieder et al. 1979; Reiley et al. 1984; Scullin et al. 1975; Suren et al. 1976; Tkaczuk 1976), osteophytes (Nachbur et al. 1979), an osteotome (May 1965; Nachbur et al. 1979), an osteosynthetic pin (Dumanian and Kelikian 1969), screws or nails (Ahlgren and Eklöf 1981; Bassett and Houck 1964; Dameron 1964; Eriksson et al. 1971; Fordyce 1968; Horton 1972; Lantin et al. 1977; Levin 1966; Meyer and Slager 1964; Wolfgang et al. 1974), intrapelvic migration of a threaded pin (Posman and Morawa 1985), or a dissection injury (Ratliff 1984)

  b) Indirect injury caused by arterial overextension and rupture (Akizuki et al. 1984)
  c) Laceration of a pseudoaneurysm with severe hemorrhage at reoperation (Bergqvist et al. 1983; Reiley et al. 1984), and on preparation of the anterior acetabular region using the Hohmann retractor (Øvrum and Dahl 1979)

2. Arterial stenosis-occlusion leading to microembolization or general distal ischemia can be caused by:
  a) Direct vessel wall injury caused by polymerization heat with successive thrombus formation (Buri 1971; Nachbur et al. 1979; Piger and Schmück 1975).

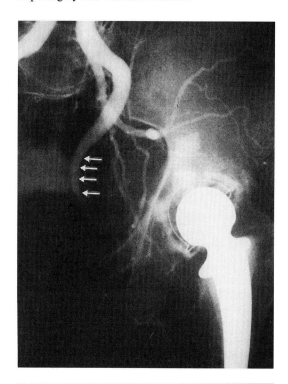

Fig. 3. Medial displacement of the external iliac artery (*arrows*) due to large thrombus-filled pseudoaneurysm after total hip replacement

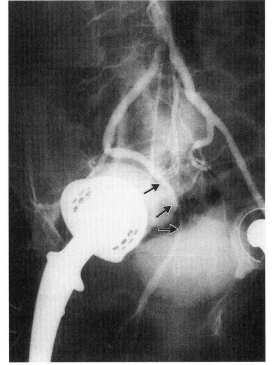

Fig. 4. Cup dislocation with medial displacement of the external iliac artery and irregularities in the wall (*arrows*). The patient had symptoms of peripheral microembolization. The diseased artery was excluded and circulation restored with femorofemoral crossover Dacron graft

b) Retractor fracture of arteriosclerotic plaques (Aust et al. 1981), mechanic occlusion with secondary thrombosis caused by cup dislocation (Fig. 4; Bergqvist et al. 1983; Thorblad 1983) or surplus of cement (Aust et al. 1981; Heyes and Aukland 1985; Hirsch et al. 1986; Nachbur et al. 1979; Neal et al. 1979; Podlaha and Schultz 1975).

c) Ligation of the common femoral artery (Bindewald et al. 1987; Salama et al. 1972) or external iliac artery (Nieder et al. 1979) because of profound bleeding, and where the anatomic topography has not been properly defined

d) Indirect injury caused by overextension with plaque or intimal rupture and development of thrombosis (Crispin and Boghemans 1980; Heyes and Aukland 1985; Jonsson et al. 1987; Nachbur et al. 1979; Schöllner and Krasemann 1975), traction with intimal avulsion (Breitenfelder and Sprangen 1973; Schöllner and Krasemann 1975), and traction causing thrombosis in the inferior epigastric artery with propagation into the iliac artery (Stubbs et al. 1986).

3. Peroperative division of important collateral arteries in patients with a borderline ischemia may cause various degrees of postoperative ischemic symptoms. Matos et al. (1979) reported on four patients, at least three of whom developed acute ischemia after total hip replacement, with rest pain and ischemic ulcerations. Angiography showed extensive arteriosclerosis with poor collateral circulation. The patients underwent reconstructive surgery.

4. Venous injuries have been reported in a much lower frequency than have arterial, the most dramatic being laceration with heavy bleeding.

Incidence

Vascular trauma after hip surgery has been described mostly after elective total hip replacement, but there have also been a number of cases after hip fracture surgery. Elective and emergency hip operations are among the most frequent orthopedic surgical procedures; moreover, both are increasing in frequency (Mannius et al. 1987). The total number of hip replacements worldwide was estimated at 350000 in 1984 (Swann 1984). From that perspective the incidence of vascular complications attributed to this type of surgery can be considered low. The increasing awareness of the problem is reflected in an editorial in the *Journal of Bone and Joint Surgery* (Ratliff 1985). Several review articles and textbooks on total hip replacement do not even mention vascular trauma as a possible complication, however (Amstutz 1970; Green 1976; Kay 1973; Lazansky 1973). In his article "Total Hip Prostheses," Müller (1970) mentioned the possibility that the tip of a Hohmann retractor might perforate the femoral artery or vein, especially if the exposure was inadequate. In publications covering altogether more than 5000 patients, no vascular injury was reported (Bergqvist et al. 1983; Boitzy and Zimmermann 1969; Coventry et al. 1974; Patterson and Brown 1972; Torgerson 1973) although Boitzy and Zimmermann (1969) mentioned that they had heard about two cases of bleeding caused by a retractor. Øvrum and Dahl (1979) as well as Breitenfelder and Spranger (1973) reported their cases after reoperations, and

Table 1. Data on 67 cases of arterial injury connected with hip surgery collected from the literature

Male patients	19	Vessel involved	
Female patients	48	External iliac artery	30
Right hip	29	Internal iliac artery	1
Left hip	38	Common femoral artery	12
Reoperation	28	Deep femoral artery	16
Indication for surgery		Medial circumflex artery	3
Osteoarthrosis	35	Superior gluteal artery	1
Hip fracture	17	Unknown	4
Rheumatoid arthritis	7		
Others	5		
Unknown	3		

Buchholtz et al. (1981) their cases with infectious complications. In our series from the General Hospital in Malmö, Sweden, there was no vascular complication among 1850 primary procedures, whereas three occurred after 250 reoperations (Bergqvist et al. 1983). Hohf (1963) sent a questionnaire to 3500 members of the American Academy of Orthopedic Surgeons. Among the 1163 replies there were 352 cases of vascular injury reported. Thirty-one of these occurred after hip surgery, one with a fatal outcome. Internal fixation of hip fracture was the most common procedure (12), followed by elective insertion of a prosthesis (8). Four cases ended with amputation. Ratliff (1984) circulated a questionnaire to 100 fellows of the British Orthopaedic Association with the aim of analyzing neurologic and vascular complications after total hip arthroplasty, and 50 and ten respectively were reported to him. The problem of vascular injuries and complications has been discussed in some recent reviews (Bergqvist et al. 1983; Nachbur et al. 1979; Ratliff 1984; Schuler and Flanigan 1987). Among 3640 cases of arterial reconstructive surgery there were 12 patients with vascular injuries after total hip replacement (Schlosser et al. 1982).

From case reports in the literature it has been possible to collect 67 cases of arterial injury (Table 1). To these can be added the 15 cases analyzed by Nachbur et al. (1979), the 12 by Schlosser et al. (1982), and the ten by Ratliff (1984), as well as a few single cases, a detailed evaluation of which is not possible. Some general points are of interest. The female and left-sided dominance is remarkable, as these differences are not seen in series of hip arthroplasty. The left-sided dominance was even more evident in cases of hip arthroplasty than in cases of hip fracture surgery. Almost half of the complications occurred during reoperations, thus indicating one real risk situation. Figure 5 shows the close anatomic relationship between the hip region and the pelvic vessels. Of the arteries involved, most of the deep femoral arterial injuries were seen after the hip fracture surgery and most of the external iliac artery injuries after hip arthroplasty.

The frequency of venous injuries seems much lower than that of arterial injuries. The first case was published by Mallory (1972). During total hip replacement a Harris reamer powered by an air drill penetrated the pelvic wall, with complete avulsion of the common iliac vein. It was ligated, and 8 months later there was no swelling of the leg. Among his 300 cases of total hip replacement, Kehr (1973)

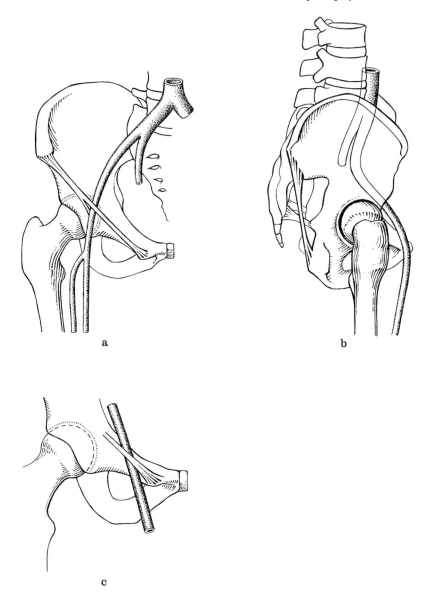

a

b

c

Fig. 5. The close pelvic relation between the acetabular/hip region and the iliacofemoral artery

had two cases of femoral vein bleeding caused by the Hohmann retractor, and Fiddian et al. (1984) described a reoperation where the femoral vein was lacerated by finger dissection. In all three cases the veins were ligated. Kehr does not mention the development of any sequelae whatsoever, whereas Fiddian et al. had infectious complications and profound swelling leading to hip disarticulation. The first vein reconstruction was reported by Nieder et al. (1979). In a patient with osteomyelitis and several reoperations, preparation of the acetabulum caused profound hemorrhage due to division of the external iliac artery and partial division of the corresponding vein. The artery was reconstructed with an interposition vein graft and the vein laceration secured with a lateral suture. In one case, pin transfixation of the external iliac vein caused hemorrhagic shock and led to vein graft replacement (Ratliff 1984). Reiley et al. (1984) mentioned a case of almost total occlusion and kinking of the external iliac vein caused by a protruding acetabular component of the prosthesis. Among 12 vascular injuries in patients with total hip replacement Schlosser et al. (1982) had two cases of venous obstruction. The displacement of iliac veins may cause secondary deep vein thrombosis and lead to cumbersome venous insufficiency (Schlosser et al. 1978). The high risk for development of deep vein thrombosis and pulmonary embolism after both elective and emergency hip surgery falls outside the scope of this discussion; nonetheless, it is a major prophylactic challenge (Bergqvist 1983). A significant proportion of these postoperative thrombi develop as a consequence of vein injury in direct relation to the orthopedic trauma.

Symptoms

Hemorrhage

There have been some cases of immediate hemorrhage during primary hip surgery (Bindewald et al. 1987; Ratliff 1984) or at reoperation (Bergqvist et al. 1983; Bindewald et al. 1987; Nieder et al. 1979; Øvrum and Dahl 1979; Reiley et al. 1984). In a few cases there has been a postoperative fall in blood pressure (Akizuki et al. 1984; Lozman and Robbins 1983; von Eggert and Huland 1974), bleeding from the wound (Akizuki et al. 1984; Aust et al. 1981; Dameron 1964; Hopkins et al. 1983), or a rapid increase in thigh circumference (Ahlgren and Eklöf 1981; May 1965) indicating ongoing bleeding. A pulsating mass is an important sign of a large arterial hemorrhage, possibly with pseudoaneurysm formation (Bassett and Houck 1964; Dumanian and Kelikian 1969; Øvrum and Dahl 1979; Suren et al. 1976). Eriksson et al. (1971) described a patient who developed an extensive intra-abdominal hemorrhage 2 years after a hip operation, from an external iliac artery pseudoaneurysm with rupture into the abdominal cavity.

Hemorrhage and Ischemia

Von Eggert and Huland (1974) described a case of immediate postoperative thigh bleeding, where the pressure from the hematoma caused ischemic symptoms as well as a drop in blood pressure. In one case, bleeding from the common femoral artery was sutured, causing stricture and ischemic symptoms, which were relieved by extirpation of the suture combined with a thrombectomy and a patch graft (Salama et al. 1972).

Ischemia

Ischemia due to impaired limb perfusion has been a common symptom (Aust et al. 1981; Breitenfelder and Spranger 1973; Crispin and Boghemans 1980; Piger and Schmück 1975; Podlaha and Schulz 1975; Neal et al. 1979; Schöllner and Krasemann 1975; Stubbs et al. 1986; Thorblad 1983). It is important to recognize local ischemia due to microembolization before extensive tissue necrosis follows (Bergqvist et al. 1983; Neal et al. 1979; Podlaha and Schulz 1975) (Fig. 4).

Neurologic Symptoms

Nerve symptoms have been caused by pressure from pseudoaneurysms on the sciatic nerve (Dorr et al. 1974), femoral nerve (Kroese and Møllerud 1975; Øvrum and Dahl 1979), or the sacral plexus (Thorblad 1983). In the last case the symptoms were rather dramatic, with paraplegia, bilateral sensibility loss, and bladder paresis.

It must be remembered, though, that nerve involvement is a frequent finding after total hip replacement, as seen from electromyographic investigations (Weber et al. 1976). Such nerve involvement is clinically evident only in rare cases, however, and the prognosis is good. Sciatic nerve neuropathy is a rare complication after hip surgery but anticoagulation increases the risk (Fleming et al. 1979; Lange 1966; Leonard 1972; Mehrotra 1967; Weber et al. 1976). One cause may be the increased pressure beneath the tightly closed fascia, and decompression is probably important in these cases.

Pain

Pain may be localized to the hip region (Aust et al. 1981; Dorr et al. 1974; Kroese and Møllerud 1975), or the patients have presented with a tender mass (Aust et al. 1981; Bergqvist et al. 1972, 1983; Fordyce 1968; Lewin 1966; Lozman and Robbins 1983; MacKenzie et al. 1983; Meyer and Slager 1964; Nieder et al. 1979; Tkaczuk 1976; Wang 1975).

Swollen Leg

Swollen leg was reported as the initial symptom in one patient in whom protusion of the prosthesis caused compression of the iliac vein as well as of the artery (Reiley et al. 1984).

Symptoms of an Arteriovenous Fistula

Cardiac insufficiency 10 years after intertrochanteric osteotomy was described by Nachbur et al. (1979). Varicose veins may develop. In one patient, bleeding at the primary operation was followed by the development of a machinery murmur, and an AV fistula between the medial circumflex femoral artery and the femoral vein was diagnosed (Ratliff 1984).

Special Problems

Especially in cases where local infectious complications have occurred, the course is often stormy, with deleterious sequelae. Amputation or disarticulation have been reported by several authors (Bergqvist et al. 1983; Dorr et al. 1974; Nachbur et al. 1979; Nieder et al. 1979, Reiley et al. 1984; Thorblad 1983), as well as fatal outcome (Nachbur et al. 1979; Nieder et al. 1979; Thorblad 1983).

Prevention

There are several factors of importance for avoiding vascular damage. When one is taking the patient's history, emphasis must be paid to arterial symptoms indicating impaired arterial circulation. A thorough examination must be made, with palpation of pulses and auscultation for bruits and, in selected cases, measurement of the ankle-brachial pressure index as well. In patients who are planned to undergo elective hip reconstruction and have symptoms or signs of lower-limb ischemia, it seems reasonable to contact and discuss the case with a vascular surgeon to decide whether or not there is an indication for prophylactic arterial reconstruction.

Anatomic knowledge is important, the pelvic vessels being situated very near to the acetabular region (Fig. 5). The possibility of profound anatomic derangements must be kept in mind in redo cases. To avoid vascular damage, strict lateral incision carries the smallest risk compared with anterolateral or posterior incisions (Ratliff 1984).

During surgery great care must be taken in using the various instruments that may cause vessel damage, such as retractors, reamers, drills, osteotomes, and screws and nails. Surplus cement, especially in the form of sharp spiculae, must be removed to eliminate the risk of subsequent vascular erosion. The role of cementation heat in inducing vascular injury has been questioned on the basis of experimental data obtained with bone cement in rabbits (Urbanyi et al. 1978). Rotation and adduction can induce overstretching injuries, especially in patients with rigid, arteriosclerotic vessels. It has been shown by venographic studies that the femoral vein is seriously distorted and at periods almost occluded during maneuvers when the femoral head is dislocated in total hip replacement (Stamatakis et al. 1977). In cases where bony support to the acetabular cup is inadequate, especially in patients with severe erosive rheumatoid arthritis, with generalized osteoporosis, or following steroid treatment, prevention of contact with the vessels can be obtained by a flanged cup or a Müller acetabular roof reinforcement (Hopkins et al. 1983).

Reoperation is a special risk situation for vascular injury, and the possibility of vascular complications must be kept in mind as a reality in such cases. Cup extraction is preferably done through a hypogastric retroperitoneal incision (similar to the incision used for kidney transplantation), making it possible to control the pelvic vessels more adequately than can be done through a lateral incision. It is also possible to remove the femoral part of the prosthesis through this hypogastric incision. In some of the cases discussed here there was a paraprosthetic infection and therefore the prosthesis was loosely connected to the femoral shaft and easily removed. At reoperation, sharp instruments should be avoided as much as possible, and care must be taken not to compress vessels between retractors and the sharp cutting edges of protruding bone, osteophytes, or cement spicules.

After all hip surgery, and especially after redo procedures, adequate observation concerning both the development of leg ischemia and signs indicating ongoing gross bleeding is a must.

Treatment

In cases of acute hemorrhage during hip surgery, placement of vascular clamps in the wound from the lateral approach is not recommended; instead, temporary hemostasis should be achieved by adequate compression. Thereafter, a hypogastric retroperitoneal incision is made to localize the pelvic vessels in an anatomically correct way, so as to make reconstruction and hemostasis possible and at the same time to guarantee adequate arterial perfusion to the extremity.

At reoperations where there is the slightest suspicion of infection, vascular reconstructions must be made either with autologous grafts or as extra-anatomic bypass procedures outside the infected field. This extra-anatomic reconstruction is usually performed as a femorofemoral crossover bypass. In most cases it is possible to construct it subcutaneously over the symphyseal region (Bergqvist et al. 1984; Bergqvist 1987; Rutherford 1985). When there is concern about the possibility of a groin infection it can be made as a transperineal graft (Hardy and Bane 1975; Taylor and Massouh 1982).

References

Ahlgren S-A, Eklöf B (1981) Femur fracture and false aneurysm. Acta Chir Scand 147:377–379
Akizuki S, Terayama K, Kobayashi S (1984) False aneurysm of the external iliac artery during total hip replacement. A case report. Arch Orthop Trauma Surg 102:210–211
Amstutz HC (1970) Complications of total hip replacement. Clin Orthop 72:123–137
Aust JC, Bredenberg CE, Murray DG (1981) Mechanisms of arterial injuries associated with total hip replacement. Arch Surg 116:345–349
Bassett FH, Houck WS (1964) False aneurysm of the profunda femoris artery after subtrochanteric osteotomy and nail-plate fixation. J Bone Joint Surg [Am] 46-A:583–585
Bergqvist D (1983) Postoperative thromboembolism. Frequency, etiology, prophylaxis. Springer, Berlin Heidelberg New York
Bergqvist D (1987) The role of extra-anatomic bypass in reoperative arterial surgery. Acta Chir Scand [Suppl] 538:61–65
Bergqvist D, Eriksson U, Grevsten S (1972) False aneurysm in the deep femoral artery as a complication of osteosynthesis of intertrochanteric femoral fracture. Acta Chir Scand 138:630–632
Bergqvist D, Carlsson ÅS, Ericsson BF (1983) Vascular complications after total hip arthroplasty. Acta Orthop Scand 54:157–163
Bergqvist D, Bergentz S-E, Ericsson BF, Helfer M, Mangell P, Takolander R (1984) Extra-anatomic vascular reconstruction in patients with aorto-iliac arteriosclerosis. Acta Chir Scand 150:205–209

Bindewald H, Ruf W, Heger W (1987) Die Verletzung der Iliacal- und Femoralgefäße – eine lebensbedrohliche Notfallsituation in der Hüftprothesenchirurgie. Chirurg 58:732–737

Boitzy A, Zimmermann H (1969) Komplikationen bei Totalprothesen der Hüfte. Arch Orthop Unfallchir 66:192–200

Breitenfelder J, Spranger M (1973) Komplikationen beim Entfernen oder Austauschen von totalen Hüftendoprothesen. Arch Orthop Unfallchir 75:56–64

Buchholtz HW, Elson RA, Engelbrecht E, Lodenkämper H, Röttger J, Siegel A (1981) Management of deep infection of total hip replacement. J Bone Joint Surg [Br] 63-B:342–353

Buri P (1971) Iatrogene Schädigung von Blutgefäßen. Helv Chir Acta 38:151–155

Coventry MB, Beckenbaugh RD, Nolan DR, Ilstrup DM (1974) 2012 total hip arthroplasties: a study of postoperative course and early complications. J Bone Joint Surg [Am] 56-A:273–284

Crispin HA, Boghemans JPM (1980) Thrombosis of the external iliac artery following total hip replacement. J Bone Joint Surg [Am] 62-A:462–464

Dameron TB (1984) False aneurysm of femoral profundus artery resulting from internal-fixation device (screw). J Bone Joint Surg [Am] 46-A:577–580

Dorr LD, Conaty JP, Kohl R, Harvey JP (1974) False aneurysm of the femoral artery following total hip surgery. J Bone Joint Surg [Am] 56-A:1059–1062

Dumanian AV, Kelikian H (1969) Vascular complications of orthopaedic surgery. J Bone Joint Surg [Am] 51-A:103–108

Eriksson I, Erikson U, Johansson H, Larsson G, Olerud S (1971) Late haemorrhage produced by arterial erosion following orthopaedic surgery. Injury 3:104–106

Fiddian NJ, Sudlow RA, Browett JP (1984) Ruptured femoral vein. A complication of the use of gentamicin beads in an infected excision arthroplasty of the hip. J Bone Joint Surg [Br] 66-B:493–494

Fleming RE, Michelsen CB, Stinchfield FE (1979) Sciatic paralysis. A complication of bleeding following hip surgery. J Bone Joint Surg [Am] 61-A:37–39

Fordyce A (1968) False aneurysm of the profunda femoris artery following nail and plate fixation of an intertrochanteric fracture. J Bone Joint Surg [Br] 50-B:141–143

Green DL (1976) Complications of total hip replacement. South Med J 69:1559–1564

Hardy JD, Bane JW (1975) Arterial injury and massive blood loss: a case report of management of pelvic gunshot injury with femoro-subscrotal-femoral bypass and 116 units of blood. Ann Surg 181:245–246

Heyes FLP, Aukland A (1985) Occlusion of the common femoral artery complicating total hip arthroplasty. J Bone Joint Surg [Br] 67-B:533–535

Hirsch SA, Robertson H, Gorniowsky M (1986) Arterial occlusion secondary to methylmethacrylate use. Arch Surg 111:204

Hohf R (1963) Arterial injuries occurring during orthopaedic operations. Clin Orthop 28:21–27

Hopkins NFG, Vanhegan JAD, Jamieson CW (1983) Iliac aneurysm after total hip arthroplasty. J Bone Joint Surg [Br] 65-B:359–361

Horton RE (1972) Arterial injuries complicating orthopaedic surgery. J Bone Joint Surg [Br] 54-B:323–327

Jonsson H, Karlström G, Lundqvist B (1987) Intimal rupture and arterial thrombosis in revisional hip arthroplasty. Case report. Acta Chir Scand 153:621–622

Kay NRM (1973) Some complications of total hip replacement. Clin Orthop 95:73–79

Kehr H (1973) Ergebnisse und Erfahrungen bei Hüftgelenkplastiken mit Totalprothesen. Monatsschr Unfallheilkd 76:49–60

Kroese A, Møllerud A (1975) Traumatic aneurysm of the common femoral artery after hip endoprosthesis. Acta Orthop Scand 46:119–122

Lange LS (1966) Lower limb palsies with hypoprothrombinaemia. Br J Med 2:93–94

Lantin F, Michel L, Vandeperre J, Lantin A (1977) Faux anévrisme de l'artère ilialque externe. Acta Chir Belg 76:347–354

Lazansky MG (1973) Complications revisited. The debit side of total hip replacement. Clin Orthop 95:96–103

Leonard MA (1972) Sciatic nerve paralysis following anticoagulation therapy. J Bone Joint
    Surg [Br] 54-B:152–153
Lewin JR (1966) The arteriographic diagnosis of pseudoaneurysm of the femoral artery re-
    sulting from an orthopedic device. Vasc Dis 3:332–334
Lozman H, Robbins H (1983) Injury to the superior gluteal artery as a complication of to-
    tal hip-replacement arthroplasty. J Bone Joint Surg [Am] 65-A:268–269
MacKenzie DB, Grobbelaar NJ, van Rensburg MNJ (1983) False aneurysm of the pro-
    funda femoris artery as a late complication of upper femoral osteotomy. S Afr J Surg
    21:255–262
Mallory TH (1972) Rupture of the common iliac vein from reaming the acetabulum during
    total hip replacement. J Bone Joint Surg [Am] 54-A:276–277
Mannius S, Mellström D, Odén A, Rundgren Å, Zetterberg C (1987) Incidence of hip frac-
    ture in western Sweden 1974–1982. Comparison of rural and urban populations. Acta
    Orthop Scand 58:38–42
Matos MH, Amstutz HA, Machleder HI (1979) Ischemia of the lower extremity after total
    hip replacement. J Bone Joint Surg [Am] 61-A:24–27
May VR (1965) Early traumatic pseudoaneurysm of the medial femoral circumflex artery
    due to the blind use of an osteotome. Clin Orthop 42:161–164
Mehrotra TN (1967) Phenindione-induced neuropathy. Br Med J 3:218
Meyer RL, Slager RF (1964) False aneurysm following subtrochanteric osteotomy. J Bone
    Joint Surg [Am] 46-A:581–582
Müller ME (1970) Total hip prostheses. Clin Orthop 72:46–68
Nachbur B, Meyer RP, Verkkala K, Zürcher R (1979) The mechanisms of severe arterial
    injury in surgery of the hip joint. Clin Orthop 141:122–133
Neal J, Wachtel TL, Garza OT, Edwards WS (1979) Late arterial embolization complicat-
    ing total hip replacement. J Bone Joint Surg [Am] 61-A:429–430
Neumann A, Berge G (1985) Arterienverletzung durch sogenannten Knochenzement. Zen-
    tralbl Chir 110:1199–1201
Nieder E, Steinbrink K, Engelbrecht E, Siegel A (1979) Verletzung von Beckengefäßen bei
    totalem Hüftgelenksersatz. Chirurg 50:780–785
Øvrum E, Dahl HK (1979) Vessel and nerve injuries complicating total hip arthroplasty.
    Arch Orthop Trauma Surg 95:267–269
Patterson FP, Brown CS (1972) The McKee-Farrar total hip replacement. Preliminary re-
    sults and complications of 368 operations performed in five general hospitals. J Bone
    Joint Surg [Am] 54-A:257–275
Piger A, Schmück L (1975) Thermische Schädigung der A. femoralis communis nach al-
    loarthroplastischem Hüftgelenkersatz. Med Monatschr 29:220–224
Podlaha J, Schulz M (1975) Arterielle Embolie nach Hüftgelenksersatz. Chirurg 46:423–
    424
Posman C, Morawa L (1985) Vascular injury from intrapelvic migration of a threaded pin.
    A case report. J Bone Joint Surg [Am] 67-A:804–806
Ratliff AHC (1984) Vascular and neurological complications. In: Lind I (ed) Complication
    of total hip replacement. Churchill Livingstone, Edinburgh, pp 18–29
Ratliff AHC (1985) Arterial injuries after total hip replacement (Editorial). J Bone Joint
    Surg [Br] 67-B:517–518
Reiley MA, Bond D, Branick RI, Wilson EH (1984) Vascular complications following total
    hip arthroplasty. Clin Orthop 186:23–28
Rutherford R (1985) Extra-anatomic bypass for aortoiliac occlusive disease. In: Kempczin-
    ski R (ed) The ischemic leg. Year Book Medical Publishers, Chicago, pp 327–337
Salama R, Stavorovsky MM, Iellin A, Weissman SL (1972) Femoral artery injury compli-
    cating total hip replacement. Clin Orthop 89:143–144
Schlosser V, Kuner EH, Spillner G (1978) Ursache von Gefäßverletzungen beim alloplasti-
    schen Hüftgelenksersatz. Chirurg 49:180–183
Schlosser V, Spillner G, Breymann T, Urbanyi B (1982) Vascular injuries in orthopaedic
    surgery. J Cardiovasc Surg (Torino) 23:323–327
Schöllner D, Krasemann P-H (1975) Akute Iliacaverschlüsse nach Austauschoperationen
    von Hüftendoprothese. Arch Orthop Unfallchir 83:305–309

Schuler J, Flanigan P (1987) Vascular repair in orthopaedic surgery of the spine and joints. In: Bergan J, Yao J (eds) Vascular surgical emergencies. Grune and Stratton, New York, pp 219–232

Scullin JP, Nelson CL, Beven EG (1975) False aneurysm of the left external iliac artery following total hip arthroplasty. Clin Orthop 113:145–149

Stamatakis JD, Kakkar VV, Sagar S, Lawrence D, Nairn D, Bentley PG (1977) Femoral vein thrombosis and total hip replacement. Br Med J 2:223–225

Stubbs DH, Dorner DB, Johnston RC (1986) Thrombosis of the iliofemoral artery during revision of a total hip replacement. J Bone Joint Surg [Am] 68-A:454–455

Suren EG, Mellmann JR, Leitz KH (1976) Gefäßkomplikationen beim alloplastischen Hüftgelenkersatz. Arch Orthop Unfallchir 85:217–224

Swann M (1984) Malignant soft-tissue tumour at the site of a total hip replacement. J Bone Joint Surg [Br] 66-B:629–631

Taylor RS, Massouh F (1982) The transperineal graft – an alternative route for femoro-femoral bypass. In: Greenhalgh R (ed) Extra-anatomic and secondary arterial reconstruction. Pitman, London, pp 237–243

Thorblad J (1983) Late vascular complication after hip arthroplasty (in Swedish). Lakartidningen 80:3817–3818

Tkaczuk H (1976) False aneurysm of the external iliac artery following hip endoprosthesis. Acta Orthop Scand 47:317–319

Torgerson WR (1973) Three years of experience with total hip replacement. Clin Orthop 95:151–157

Urbanyi B, Hanck P, Matthias K, Böhm N, Schlosser V (1978) Experimentelle Untersuchung zur Frage der Gefäßschädigung durch Knochenzement (Palacos). Langenbecks Arch Chir 346:47–52

von Eggert A, Huland H (1974) Gefäßverletzung bei Osteosynthesen am proximalen Femurschaft. Zentralbl Chir 99:946–950

Wang C-J (1975) False aneurysm of the profundus femoral artery following nail-plate fixation for intertrochanteric fracture of the hip. J Med Soc NJ 72:623

Weber ER, Daube JR, Coventry MB (1976) Peripheral neuropathies associated with total hip arthroplasty. J Bone Joint Surg [Am] 58-A:60–69

Wolfgang GL, Barnes WT, Hendricks GL (1974) False aneurysm of the profunda femoris artery resulting from nail-plate fixation of intertrochanteric fracture. Clin Orthop 100:143–150

Vascular Injuries During Lumbar Disk Surgery

Types of Injury

An analysis of reported cases reveal five main types of injury incurred during lumbar disk surgery:
1. Immediate hemorrhage
    a) From an artery (Alvarez et al. 1987; Ansvarsnämnden 1972, 1978; Birkeland and Taylor 1969; Boyd and Farha 1965; Brewster et al. 1979; Buri 1971; Franzini et al. 1987; Freeman 1961; Hohf 1963; Jue-Denis et al. 1984; Mack 1956; Mills et al. 1986; Moore and Cohen 1968; Morisi and Terragni 1967; Piger and Scherer 1973; Salander et al. 1984; Schlosser et al. 1982; Seeley et al. 1954; Shumacker et al. 1961; Stevenson et al. 1981)
    b) From a vein (Alvarez et al. 1987; Freeman 1961; Mack 1956; Moore and Cohen 1968; Stevenson et al. 1981)
2. Arteriovenous fistula (Fig. 1; Areskog et al. 1964; Boyd and Farha 1965; Chiache et al. 1960; Davies 1969; DeBakey et al. 1958; Dumanian and Keli-

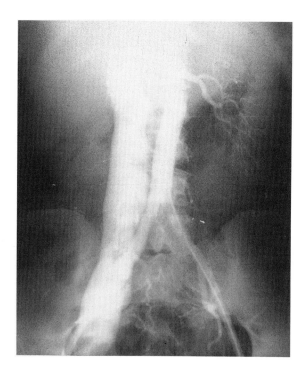

Fig. 1. A 43-year-old woman had 2 years previously undergone disk surgery with an extensive intraoperative venous hemorrhage. During a clinical check-up in connection with a common cold a bruit was heard and cardiac insufficiency appeared imminent. Angiogram shows a large fistula between the right common iliac artery and vein. Preoperative heart minute volume was 13 l; this decreased to 8 l immediately after closure of the fistula

kian 1969; Evans 1974; Fortune 1956; Glass and Ilgenfritz 1954; Görömbey et al. 1984; Harbison 1954; Hardin and Allen 1958; Hildreth and Turcke 1977; Hofmann et al. 1974; Hohf 1963; Holscher 1948; Horton 1961, 1972; Hufnagel et al. 1961; Jarstfer and Rich 1976; Linton and White 1945; Mack 1956; Marks et al. 1971; May et al. 1981; Quigley and Stoney 1985; Rossi et al. 1974; Salander et al. 1984; Saldino et al. 1971; Schlosser et al. 1982; Schreiber et al. 1967; Smith et al. 1957; Solonen 1964; Spittell et al. 1963; Staple and Friedenberg 1965; Staab et al. 1968; Steinberg et al. 1961; Sze et al. 1960; Taylor and Williams 1962; Ueda et al. 1964; Vargas et al. 1964; Wajszczuk et al. 1969)
3. Pseudoaneurysm in combination with arteriovenous fistula (Brewster et al. 1979; Hildreth and Turcke 1977; May et al. 1981; Quigley and Stoney 1985; Saldino et al. 1971; Shumacker et al. 1961; Smith and Killen 1973; Vargas et al. 1964)
4. Pseudoaneurysm without fistulization (Mills et al. 1986; Salander et al. 1984, two cases; Seeley et al. 1954)
5. Partial avulsion with development of thrombosis (Stokes 1968)

Incidence

In 1934, Mixter and Barr described diskectomy in the treatment of prolapsed lumbar intervertebral disks compressing the nerve roots. About 10 years later, the first vascular complication after such an operation was reported by Linton and White from Boston (1945), in the form of an arteriovenous fistula between the right common iliac artery and vein. Half a year after the disk operation the patient developed cardiac incompensation and was treated with a two-stage surgical procedure: first sympathectomy of the first to the fourth lumbar ganglions and then ligation of the common iliac artery and vein. Except for a probably pulmonary embolism, the patient had no sequelae. The 10-year delay between the first disk operation and the first reported vascular complication is considered to have been due to a less radical surgical attitude towards the prolapsed disk in those years.

The true frequency of vascular complications in connection with lumbar disk surgery is not known. Harbison (1954) sent letters to 100 surgeons belonging to the American Surgical Association and received reliable information concerning 25 injures to major blood vessels. These cases were reviewed together with five further cases. The mortality was found to be extremely high at 61%. Nine of the cases involved arteriovenous fistulae, two of which had a fatal outcome (22%); thus the mortality was considerably lower than among the rest of the patients.

DeSaussure (1959) sent 3027 questionnaires to 739 neurosurgeons and 2288 members of the American Orthopedic Association and got an "excellent response." One hundred and six vascular injuries in connection with lumbar disk surgery were reported. Most commonly, the injuries were caused by the pituitary rongeur, in rare cases by a curet. Also in this series the mortality was high (46%), the lowest rate being for cases of late arteriovenous fistulas (16%). Apropos of frequency, DeSaussure quoted results from a series of 6000 operations in Memphis where only one unspecified vascular injury was seen, but with a fatal outcome.

Hohf (1963) also sent a questionnaire to 3500 members of the American Academy of Orthopedic Surgeons. He chose the most qualified surgeons in the field or, in other words, those who were least likely to have complications. His aim was to survey arterial injuries occurring during all types of orthopedic operations. He received 1163 answers, reporting 352 injuries which it was possible to analyze; 59 were related to herniated disk surgery. Late complications were five arteriovenous fistulae and one pseudoaneurysm, the others being emergency cases. The mortality was around 25%.

Holscher (1968) updated and reviewed the literature and added 12 unpublished cases, unfortunately not with enough details to make a further analysis possible. At any rate, there were six deaths, all in immediate connection with the operation. Among 3640 arterial reconstructive procedures Schlosser et al. (1982) had two cases of arterial injury caused by resection of a herniated disk. It seems certain that although many cases remain unpublished, the frequency is low at probably less than 1‰.

The vessels are the structures with the closest anatomic relation to the vertebral column, but there are also reports of injuries to organs such as the intestine (Birkeland and Taylor 1969, 1970; Smith and Estridge 1964) and the ureter (Sandoz and Hodges 1965; Moore and Cohen 1968; Kern et al. 1969). Over the years there have been several published reviews of the problem (Harbison 1954; Hildreth and Turcke 1977; Jarstfer and Rich 1976; Montorsi and Ghiringhelli 1973; Schuler and Flanigan 1987; Stokes 1968).

Immediate Hemorrhagic Complications

In 26 patients (17 male, eight female, one gender not reported) described in the literature the vascular complication was of a nonfistular type, that is, bleeding was closely related to the lumbar disk operation. The L4–5 interspace dominated (20 cases), followed by L5–S1 (6), L3–4 (1), and two unspecified. Figure 2 shows

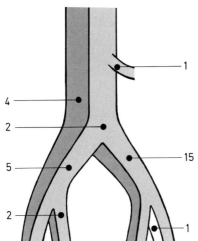

Fig. 2. Location of immediate hemorrhagic complications after lumbar disk surgery (survey of published cases)

the location of the 29 injuries. In four patients there were injuries to both an artery and a vein, but a fistula had not formed at the time of reoperation. Two patients were not operated on and died, one 11 h postoperatively with injury to the left common iliac artery and inferior vena cava (Freeman 1961), the other 9 h postoperatively with lacerations of the inferior vena cava (Mack 1956). Another patient died on the operating table during attempted hemostasis of a laceration of the right internal iliac artery (Mack 1956). One patient died postoperatively because of hypovolemic shock (Ansvarsnämnden 1978). In one case, an immediate exploratory laparatomy was done, but as the large retroperitoneal hematoma did not expand, no further identification of the cause of bleeding was made (Seeley et al. 1954). About 1 week later a pseudoaneurysm from an injury of the common iliac artery was reconstructed with a homograft, and after 30 days another pseudoaneurysm developed in the reconstructed area. Ligation with no further reconstruction was made, and there were no further sequelae. Further complications observed involved one patient with occlusion after reconstruction of a lacerated left common iliac artery with development of claudication (Birkeland and Taylor 1969), one patient with concomitant ureteral injury and meningitis who survived (Moore and Cohen 1968), one patient with a false aneurysm after reconstruction (Salander et al. 1984), and one patient with a swollen leg after ligation of the left common iliac vein (Stevenson et al. 1981).

Arteriovenous Fistula

There are 68 reports in the literature (42 male patients, 23 female patients, and three of unreported gender) from which it is possible to obtain data for detailed analysis. In eleven of the cases there had been more than one lumbar operation for disk problems. Table 1 shows the level of disk surgery. Table 2 shows data from the

Table 1. Level of disk surgery performed in 68 cases reported in the literature

	No. of lesions
L 3–4	5
L 4–5	37
L 5–S 1	13
Unknown	17

Table 2. Early symptoms in connection with the disk operation in 68 cases with arteriovenous fistulae reported in the literature

Profuse peroperative bleeding	17
Peroperative fall in blood pressure	13
Postoperative fall in blood pressure	3
Unilateral leg cyanosis	1
Back and/or abdominal problems	8
Postoperative fall in hematocrit	5

disk operation. Injury to a major vessel is usually indicated by a sudden gush of blood from the disk space. This is a most important sign. In many instances this bleeding can be controlled adequately by packing, but such patients should be carefully monitored, early on for continued bleeding and later for the development of an arteriovenous fistula. The median time from disk surgery to operation for the fistula was 6 months, with a range of 1 day to 9 years. Some of the patients lived with severe heart failure for a long time before the correct diagnosis was established. The dominating symptom by far was high-output congestive heart failure (Table 3). A common debut symptom, before heart failure developed, was swelling of one or both legs. Pulmonary embolism was reported by Harbison (1954) and was thereafter described in another three cases (Solonen 1964; Brewster et al. 1979; May et al. 1981). Figure 3 shows the location of the fistulae, most of them in immediate relation to the aortic bifurcation.

The diagnosis is difficult and often delayed. One of the case reports (Fortune 1956) deals with a rather typical patient (a 36-year-old man) in whom the fistula was not detected until autopsy after death of cardiac failure.

Table 3. Dominating symptoms and signs in 68 patients with arteriovenous fistula

Heart failure	42
Abdominal pain	9
Leg swelling	6
Pulmonary embolism	3
Pulsating mass	1
Machinery murmur in patients with	
Heavy blood loss	1
Cardiomegaly	1
Tachycardia	1
Machinery murmur on auscultation	4
in patients with various non-related symptoms	

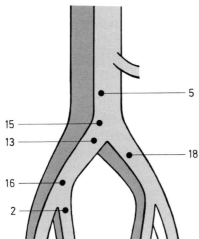

Fig. 3. Location of arteriovenous fistulae after lumbar disk surgery (survey of published cases)

Prevention

Knowledge of normal anatomic relationships is important, to prevent this type of injury (Figs. 4, 5). The aortic bifurcation is located somewhat to the left of the midline and, in 70–80% of cases, at the level of the L4–5 interspace and close to the anterior longitudinal ligament. The confluence of the iliac veins is somewhat more caudally situated, the left common iliac vein between the right common iliac artery and the body of L5. When the anterior ligament is perforated during disk

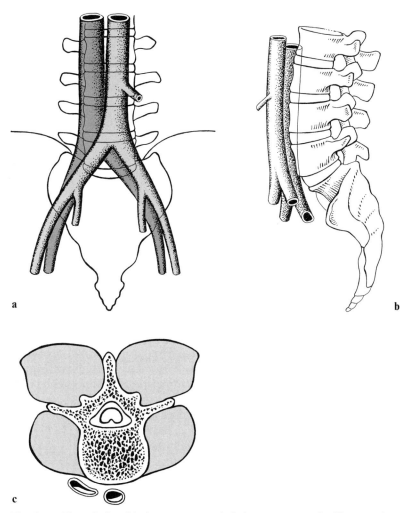

a   b

c

Fig. 4 a–c. The relationship between aorta, inferior vena cava, the iliac vessels, and the lumbar vertebrae. The aorta bifurcates at the lower border of L4 or at the disk between L4 and L5 in the majority of cases, although in women often somewhat more distally. The confluence between the iliac veins to form the inferior vena cava is directly distal to and to the right of the aortic bifurcation. Disks L3–L4 and L4–L5 and occasionally L5–S1 are in closest relationship to the vessels

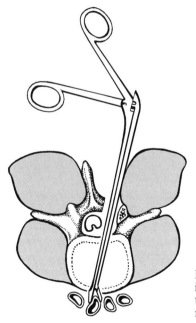

Fig. 5. A cross section through the disk L4–L5 showing the pituitary rongeur penetrating the disk and
the arterial longitudinal ligament and damaging the
right iliac artery

surgery the distance to the vessels is very short. The close topographic relation
during surgery has been beautifully demonstrated with intraoperative angiographies by Nilsonne and Hakelius (1965). Sharp instruments such as pituitary
rongeurs and curets must be handled with the utmost care, but the majority of
injuries occur in spite of the fact that the operative procedure is performed by an
experienced surgeon (Schuler and Flanigan 1987). The surgeon must be con-
stantly aware of contacting the vertebral bodies with the tip of the rongeur. Exploration of the disk space must be done with the instrument closed. When remaining disk fragments are present the instrument is slightly open and care must
be taken to avoid further penetration at this stage. Even using normal operative
force it is possible to penetrate the vertebral body with these instruments (Marks
et al. 1971). The use of such instruments to measure distances cannot be recommended. Degenerative processes of the annulus fibrosis and the anterior ligament
may make those tissues more vulnerable and more easily penetrated. There may
also be true fissures in the anterior annulus (Leavens and Bradford 1953). Hyper-
trophic spurs, spondylolysis, spondylolisthesis, and other anomalies may increase
the risk of vascular injuries. Degenerative joint disease may cause scarring and
a relative fixation of the vessels. Reoperation seems to be a special risk factor. The
position of the patient with pressure on the abdominal contents also tends to press
the vessels toward the vertebral column. Simmons and Wilber (1986) have discussed technical surgical points that should be considered in order to avoid vascular
damage.

Treatment

As already stated, the injury can cause acute hemorrhagic symptoms as well as a more gradual development of symptoms because of an arteriovenous fistula. When both arteries and veins are injured, the lowest resistance is obviously in the venous system compared with the surrounding tissue, and this is why even rather large holes in the vessels give rise to fistulization rather than to immediate exsanguination. In a few cases there has been a combination of bleeding into the tissue, creating a spurious aneurysm, and fistulization.

During the primary disk operation profuse bleeding should always be a warning sign, as should intra- or postoperative pressure drops where no other obvious explanation is at hand. It is very dangerous to blame the blood pressure drop in this situation on anesthesiologic complications or myocardial dysfunction without considering the possibility of a vascular injury. Packing of the wound may stop the posterior bleeding and at the same time lull the surgeon into a false feeling of security. In cases of acute hemorrhage rapid and correct handling is necessary if death is to be avoided. The patient must be moved rapidly to a supine position and an exploratory laparatomy should be done immediately. In the postoperative period abdominal pain and paralysis should also raise the suspicion of vascular damage with retroperitoneal hemorrhage. In such patients, provided their circulation is stable, computerized tomography would probably be of diagnostic value. More frequent use of a stethoscope to listen for abdominal machinery murmur could often give a correct diagnosis before severe symptoms of heart failure occur.

Heart failure is rare when fistulas have a diameter of less than 10 mm (Hildreth and Turcke 1977). In many of the published cases there has been a rather long diagnostic delay between the common debut symptom of swollen legs and the more severe symptoms of heart failure. A machinery murmur centered in the region of the umbilicus together with a thrill in patients who have undergone disk surgery are practically pathognomonic. From a surgical strategic point a view, angiography is of value to show the exact location of the fistula and to show if it is combined with a pseudoaneurysm. Before operation of the fistula the patients must be in optimal condition cardiologically.

In case of bleeding during surgery, the cause must be localized and a reconstruction done. Today it cannot be considered lege artis to do primary ligation of the vessels; reconstruction must be the aim.

Several surgical methods have been used to solve the problem of closing the fistula, from four-vessel ligation with or without sympathectomy in the early days to various types of reconstruction. In the literature reviewed two patients died postoperatively, one because of respiratory arrest (Marks et al. 1971) and one because of a probably aortoenteric fistula after ligation of the aorta and the vena cava (Spittell et al. 1963). In two cases postoperative pulmonary embolism occurred (Linton and White 1945; Vargas et al. 1964) and in one a nonfatal myocardial infarction (Saldino et al. 1971). Leg swelling was noted in three patients, one of whom had a deep vein thrombosis diagnosed. In two of the seven patients in whom the artery was ligated moderate intermittent claudication developed, in no case gangrene. In case of fistulas all four vessels should be mobilized and se-

cured. The dissection may be difficult, as the vessel injuries are located pos-
teriorly. With some injuries to the inferior vena cava it may be easier to make an
anterior venotomy and repair the posterior lesion through the vena cava. Both
the artery and the vein should be reconstructed, if necessary with an arterial graft.
It is not enough to ligate the fistula; it must be divided. Otherwise there is a high
risk of recurrence. If there is a concomitant pseudoaneurysm, care must be taken
not to embolize thrombotic contents during the surgical manipulation, causing
a pulmonary embolism. During exploratory laparatomy other injuries should be
looked for as well.

References

Alvarez H, Cazarez J, Hernandez A (1987) An alternative repair of major vascular injury
    inflicted during lumbar disk surgery. Surgery 101:505–507
Ansvarsnämnden (1972) Acquittal decision in a case of Lex Maria (in Swedish). Lakartid-
    ningen 69:3186–3187
Ansvarsnämnden (1978) Rare complication of lumbar disk surgery (in Swedish). Lakartid-
    ningen 75:2486–2487
Areskog N-H, Löf B, Nylander G, Sundquist O, Thorén L (1964) Arteriovenous fistula be-
    tween the common iliac artery and vein. Vasc Dis 1:113–118
Birkeland IW, Taylor TKF (1969) Major vascular injuries in lumbar disc surgery. J Bone
    Joint Surg [Br] 51-B:4–19
Birkeland IW, Taylor TKF (1970) Bowel injuries coincident to lumbar disk surgery: a re-
    port of four cases and a review of the literature. J Trauma 10:163–168
Boyd DP, Farha GJ (1965) Arteriovenous fistula and isolated vascular injuries secondary
    to intervertebral disk surgery. Ann Surg 161:524–531
Brewster DC, May ARL, Darling RC, Abbott WM, Moncure AC (1979) Variable mani-
    festations of vascular injury during lumbar disk surgery. Arch Surg 114:1026–1030
Buri P (1971) Iatrogene Schädigung von Blutgefäßen. Helv Chir Acta 38:151–155
Chiache K, Tsuji H, Schobinger R, Kniesel J, Cooper P (1960) Arteriovenous fistula be-
    tween the common iliac vessels. Report of a case corrected surgically. Arch Surg
    80:258–261
Davies JMC (1969) Ilio-iliac arteriovenous fistula following laminectomy. Clin Radiol
    20:103–104
DeBakey ME, Cooley DA, Morris GC, Collins H (1958) Arteriovenous fistula involving
    the abdominal aorta: report of four cases with successful repair. Ann Surg 147:646–
    658
DeSaussure RL (1959) Vascular injury coincident to disk surgery. J Neurosurg 16:222–
    229
Dumanian A, Kelikian H (1969) Vascular complications of orthopaedic surgery. J Bone
    Joint Surg [Am] 51-A:103–108
Evans WE (1974) Arteriovenous fistula following disc surgery. Vasc Surg 8:33–35
Fortune C (1956) Arterio-venous fistula of the left common iliac artery and vein. Med J
    Aust 1:660–661
Franzini M, Altana P, Annessi V, Lodini V (1987) Iatrogenic vascular injuries following
    lumbar disc surgery. Case report and review of the literature. J Cardiovasc Surg
    (Torino) 28:727–730
Freeman DG (1961) Major vascular complications of lumbar disc surgery. West J Surg Ob-
    stet Gynecol 69:175–177
Glass BA, Ilgenfritz HC (1954) Arteriovenous fistula secondary to operation for ruptured
    intervertebral disc. Ann Surg 140:122–127
Görömbey Z, Gömöry A, Békáassy SM (1984) Iatrogenic aortocaval fistula secondary to
    intervertebral disc surgery. Acta Chir Scand 150:585–588

Harbison SP (1954) Major vascular complications of intervertebral disc surgery. Ann Surg 140:342–438
Hardin CA, Allen M (1958) Arteriovenous fistula. J Kans Med Soc 59:93–95
Hildreth DH, Turcke DA (1977) Postlaminectomy arteriovenous fistula. Surgery 81:512–520
Hofmann KT, Simonis G, Männl HFK, Koch B (1974) Iatrogene Verletzungen der großen Gefäße und am Herzen. Muench Med Wochenschr 116:975–982
Hohf R (1963) Arterial injuries occurring during orthopaedic operations. Clin Orthop 28:21–37
Holscher EC (1948) Vascular complication of disk surgery. J Bone Joint Surg [Am] 30-A:968–970
Holscher EC (1985) Vascular and visceral injuries during lumbar-disk surgery. J Bone Joint Surg [Am] 50-A:383–393
Horton RE (1961) Arteriovenous fistula following operation for prolapsed intervertebral disk. Br J Surg 49:77–80
Horton RE (1972) Arterial injuries complicating orthopaedic surgery. J Bone Joint Surg [Br] 54-B:323–327
Hufnagel CA, Walsh BJ, Conrad PW (1961) Iliac-caval arteriovenous fistula following operation for herniated disc. Angiology 12:579–582
Jarstfer BS, Rich NM (1976) The challenge of arteriovenous fistula formation following disk surgery: a collective review. J Trauma 16:726–733
Jue-Denis P, Kieffer E, Benhamon M, de Thoai H, Richard T, Natali J (1984) Traumatismes des vaisseaux abdominaux après chirurgie de la hernie discale. Rev Chir Orthop 70:141–145
Kern HB, Barnes W, Malamant M (1969) Lumbar laminectomy and associated ureteral injury. J Urol 102:675–677
Leavens M, Bradford K (1953) Ruptured intervertebral disc. Report of a case with a defect in the anterior annulus fibrosus. J Neurosurg 10:544–546
Linton RR, White PD (1945) Arteriovenous fistula between the right common iliac artery and the inferior vena cava. Report of a case of its occurrence following an operation for a ruptured intervertebral disk with cure by operation. Arch Surg 50:6–13
Mack JR (1956) Major vascular injuries incident to intervertebral disk surgery. Am Surg 22:752–763
Marks C, Weiner SN, Reydman M (1971) Arteriovenous fistula secondary to intervertebral disc surgery. J Cardiovasc Surg (Torino) 12:417–424
May ARL, Brewster DC, Darling RC, Browse NL (1981) Arteriovenous fistula following lumbar disc surgery. Br J Surg 69:41–43
Mills J, Wiedeman J, Robinson J (1986) Minimizing mortality and morbidity from iatrogenic arterial injuries: the need for early recognition and prompt repair. J Vasc Surg 4:22–27
Mixter WJ, Barr JS (1934) Rupture of the intervertebral disk with involvement of the spinal cord. N Engl J Med 211:210–215
Montorsi W, Ghiringhelli C (1973) Genesis, diagnosis and treatment of vascular complications after intervertebral disk surgery. Int Surg 58:233–235
Moore CA, Cohen CA (1968) Combined arterial, venous, and uretral injury complicating lumbar disk surgery. Am J Surg 115:574–577
Morisi M, Terragni R (1967) Una gravissima complicanza dell' intervento per ernia discale lombare: la lesione dei grossi vasi retroperitoneali. Arch Orthop 80:307–316
Nilsonne U, Hakelius A (1965) On vascular injury in lumbar disc surgery. Acta Orthop Scand 35:329–337
Piger A, Scherer H (1973) Iatrogene Verletzung der Arteria iliaca communis: eine seltene Komplikation der Diskus-Prolaps-Operation im Lumbalbereich. Vasa 2:152–155
Quigley T, Stoney R (1985) Arteriovenous fistulas following lumbar laminectomy: the anatomy defined. J Vasc Surg 2:828–833
Rossi P, Carillo FJ, Alfidi RJ (1974) Iatrogenic arteriovenous fistulas. Radiology 111:47–51

Salander JM, Youkey JR, Rich NM, Olson DW, Clagett GP (1984) Vascular injury related to lumbar disk surgery. J Trauma 24:628–631

Saldino RM, White AA, Palubinskas AJ (1971) Arteriovenous fistula, a complication of lumbar disk surgery. Diagn Radiol 98:565–567

Sandoz J, Hodges CV (1965) Ureteral injury incident to lumbar disc operation. J Urol 93:687–689

Schlosser V, Spillner G, Breymann T, Urbanyi B (1982) Vascular injuries in orthopaedic surgery. J Cardiovasc Surg (Torino) 23:323–327

Schreiber MH, Wolma FJ, Morettin LB (1967) Angiographic findings in arteriovenous fistulas following lumbar disk surgery. Am J Roentgenol Radium Ther Nucl Med 101:957–960

Schuler J, Flanigan P (1987) Vascular repair in orthopaedic surgery of the spine and joints. In: Bergan J, Yao J (eds) Vascular surgical emergencies. Grune and Stratton, New York, pp 219–232

Seeley SF, Hughes CW, Jahnke EJ (1954) Major vessel damage in lumbar disc operation. Surgery 35:421–429

Shumacker HB, King H, Campbell R (1961) Vascular complications from disc operation. J Trauma 1:177–185

Simmons E, Wilber G (1986) Complications of spinal surgery for discogenic disease and spondylolisthesis. In: Epps C (ed) Complications in orthopedic surgery. Lippincott, Philadelphia

Smith VM, Hughes CW, Joy RJT, Mattingly TW (1957) High-output circulatory failure due to arteriovenous fistula. Arch Intern Med 100:833

Smith RA, Estridge MN (1964) Bowel perforation following lumbar-disc surgery. Report of a case with a review of the literature. J Bone Joint Surg [Am] 46-A:826–828

Smith RF, Killen DA (1973) Arteriovenous fistula and chronic congestive heart failure following intervertebral disk surgery. South Med J 66:1301–1303

Solonen KA (1964) Arteriovenous fistula as a complication of operation for prolapsed disk. Acta Orthop Scand 34:159–166

Spittell JA, Palumbo PJ, Love JG, Ellis FH (1963) Arteriovenous fistula complicating lumbar-disk surgery. N Engl J Med 268:1162–1166

Staab RC, Stoever WW, Baldwin W, Hickman M (1968) Arteriovenous fistula complicating lumbar disc surgery: report of a case. J Am Osteopath Assoc 67:1379–1381

Staple TW, Friedenberg MJ (1965) Ilio-iliac arteriovenous fistula following intervertebral disc surgery. Clin Radiol 16:248–250

Steinberg I, Glenn F, Carver ST, Lukas DS (1961) Angiographic and hemodynamic studies of a postlaminectomy iliac arterial inferior vena caval fistula. Am J Med 31:310–317

Stevenson IM, Littler J (1981) Iliac vessel injury complicating lumbar laminectomy. J R Coll Surg Edinb 26:187–188

Stokes J (1968) Vascular complications of disk surgery. J Bone Joint Surg [Am] 50-A:394–399

Sze K, Tsuji H, Schobinger R, Kneisel J, Cooper P (1960) Arteriovenous fistula between the common iliac vessels. Report of a case corrected surgically. Arch Surg 80:258–261

Taylor H, Williams E (1962) Arteriovenous fistula following disk surgery. Br J Surg 50:47–50

Ueda H, Tagawa H, Saito S, Nakahara K (1964) A case of arteriovenous fistula following lumbar-disk surgery (in Japanese). J Jpn Soc Intern Med 53:1046–1050

Vargas CZ, Abugattas R, Santa Maria E, Battilana G, Guibovich C (1964) Arteriovenous fistula between the common right iliac artery and the inferior vena cava incident to intervertebral disk surgery (report of two cases). J Cardiovasc Surg (Torino) 5:392–400

Wajszczuk WJ, Mowry FM, Whitcomb JG (1969) Arteriovenous fistula – a complication of surgery of intervertebral disc. Rocky Mt Med J 66:37–39

Vascular Injuries During Gynecologic Surgery

Types of Injury

Injuries that may occur during gynecologic laparotomy are (a) laceration with bleeding from an artery and/or a vein, (b) arterial occlusion leading to ischemia, and (c) arteriovenous fistula. Those that may occur during gynecologic laparoscopy are (a) laceration of an artery or a vein with bleeding and (b) arterial occlusion with ischemia.

Incidence

In gynecologic pelvic operations the close topographic relation to important vessels is obvious. It would not be surprising if there were an increasing frequency of vascular injuries with an increasing aggressiveness in pelvic cancer surgery. However, the incidence of vascular injuries during gynecologic laparotomies is largely unknown, and the few case reports that exist probably underestimate the problem. One reason could be that the vascular problems are solved during surgery and therefore not reported. A questionnaire to Swedish clinics undertaking gynecologic surgery focused on the incidence of vascular injury and analyzed types of injuries for the period 1979–1983 (Bergqvist and Bergqvist 1987). The response rate was high, but the figures obtained are probably still low because of faulty registration of injuries. In Table 1 the calculated incidence is shown. Among 87 iatrogenic injuries reported at the Walter Reed Army Medical Center in Washington, four occurred during gynecologic surgery (Rich et al. 1974).

Much more is written about complications to laparoscopy than to laparotomy, but the frequency of major vascular injuries is obviously very low. However, laparoscopically induced injuries dramatically change the course for the patients, with prolonged hospitalization, added morbidity, and risk of a fatal out-

Table 1. Incidence of major vascular injuries during gynecologic surgery in Sweden from 1979 to 1983. (After Bergqvist and Bergqvist (1987), based on a countrywide questionnaire with a response rate of 98%)

	No. of operations	No. of patients injured	Incidence per 10 000 operations
Laparoscopy	75 035	7	0.93
Laparotomy	81 889	7	0.76
Vaginal operation	30 750	1	0.33

Table 2. Major vascular injuries during laparoscopy based on survey of the literature

	No. of laparoscopies	No. of major vascular injuries	Frequency (%)
Schneller et al. (1982)	1 613	0	0
De Boer and Hutchins (1975)	643	2	0.31
Duignan et al. (1972)	1 000	0	0
Moldin and Jacobson (1984)	1 135	0	0
Frenkel et al. (1981)	2 757	1	0.04
Lübke (1977)	2 800	4	0.14
Corson and Bolognese (1972)	1 545	0	0
Nilsen and Jerve (1976)	1 168	0	0
Havemann et al. (1977)	2 700	0	0
Buytaert and Meulyzer	892	0	0
	15 953	7	0.04

come. Unfortunately, even papers dealing with complications to laparoscopy do not always define the type of vascular injury, and a detailed analysis is therefore impossible. In Table 2, data are collected from some publications, the frequency being much lower than the one shown in Table 1 from Sweden, where an active search for the cases was undertaken. Lacerations of vessels in the mesentery, omentum, or mesosalpinx are not included in the table (Courly et al. 1973; Esposito and Rubino 1974; Esposito 1973). Loffer and Pent (1975) and Frangenheim (1971) discussed lesions to major vessels as a possibility but did not give any details. Mintz (1977) reviewed 99 204 laparoscopies: There were 123 laparotomies necessitated by various complications with four fatal outcomes, all after bowel injuries. There were 34 major vessel injuries, 20 from the insufflating needle, 11 from the trocar, and three from the probing needle. Penfield (1977) sent a questionnaire concerning major vessel injuries to 25 of the most knowledgeable and experienced laparoscopists in the United States, Canada, Great Britain, and Holland. He received replies from 19, 12 of whom described 19 cases. Unfortunately, the total number of laparoscopies performed among which these injuries occurred is not given. The remaining seven responders had seen major vascular injuries in some 30 000 laparoscopies.

Injuries giving rise to intraoperative or immediately postoperative hemorrhagic problems are probably severely underreported, and the true incidence can be established only in a prospective study.

Vascular Injuries During Laparoscopy

There are altogehter 56 patients described in the literature who incurred injuries during laparoscopy. The indication for laparoscopy was not given in 46% of the reports. In the others, sterilization dominated (35%), followed by investigation for ovarian tumors (9.6%) and fertility (5.8%), Except for three injuries to mesenteric arteries (Bartsich and Dillon 1981; Penfield 1977; Rust et al. 1980; Sirinek and Levine 1985) and one to splenic vessels (Fear 1968), the injuries have been located in the aortoiliac region. In two patients delayed symptoms occurred. In one there was bleeding from necrotic defects in the right common iliac artery and vein 3 months after the laparoscopic procedure (Bistler et al. 1980). In the other, successively increasing sciatic pain following ovarian biopsy led to the discovery of a pseudo-aneurysm of the superior gluteal artery. Embolization was tried without effect, but occlusion was succesfully managed with 48-h Fogarty balloon inflation of the bleeding artery. In only three cases were there isolated venous injuries (Cohen 1971; Parewijck et al. 1979; Penfield 1977), and in four there were venous and arterial injuries in combination (Bistler et al. 1980; Katz et al. 1979; McDonald et al. 1978; Bergan 1987). In one of the vein injuries carbon dioxide was insufflated into the left common iliac vein, resulting in a fatal gas embolism (Parewijck et al. 1979), a complication which is very rare; Minth (1977) collected data from 100000 laparoscopies and described only three cases of fatal gas embolism.

Vessels Damaged

Injury to the arterial system most frequently involved the aorta (Fig. 1; Bistler et al. 1980; Erkrath et al. 1979; Katz et al. 1979; Kurzel and Edinger 1983; Lynn et al. 1982; McDonald et al. 1978; Penfield 1977; Peterson et al. 1982; Shin 1982; Lübke 1977; Chapin et al. 1980). In one case the internal iliac artery was damaged (Buri 1971), in one the right external iliac artery (Lignitz et al. 1985), and in the remaining the common iliac arteries with predominance of the right (Bergqvist and Bergqvist 1987; Bistler et al. 1980; DeBoer and Hutchins 1975; Frenkel et al. 1981; Heinrich et al. 1985; Hulka et al. 1973; Katz et al. 1979; McDonald et al. 1978; Penfield 1977; Rust et al. 1980; Lübke 1977; Bergan 1987).

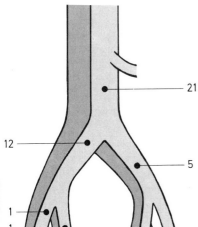

21

12

5

1

1

Fig. 1. Location of 40 arterial injuries induced during laparoscopy, from a literature survey. Of the 56 reported cases, three were mesenteric, one was splenic, and ten were without known anatomical location. Two of the injuries were of a delayed type

Symptoms and Diagnosis

In one case the diagnosis was missed altogether; the patient died in hemorrhagic shock and the damage was detected at autopsy (Peterson et al. 1982). All the remaining 55 patients were operated on; the bleeding was localized and in most cases managed with a simple suture. However, seven patients died postoperatively, giving a mortality of 13.2%, and one patient survived after profound shock but lived as a cerebral vegetable. The bleeding was mostly discovered during the laparoscopic procedure and led to immediate laparotomy, but a few patients developed signs of bleeding in the recovery room. There were three moments during laparoscopy when injuries occurred – insertion of the insufflation needle, insertion of the trocar, and use of biopsy forceps. One case is illustrated in Fig. 2.

Vascular Injuries During Laparotomy

Acute Problems

Boontje (1981) mentioned two cases of injury occurring during hysterectomy, probably of the external iliac arteries. Lord et al. (1958) reported in detail on a patient with severe hemorrhage during hysterectomy, where both the internal iliac arteries were ligated. Moreover, the left common iliac artery was severely lacerated, leading to ischemic symptoms which were relieved by implantation of the left common iliac artery into the right one. Heinrich et al. (1985), without giving any details, reported five vascular injuries during pelvic surgery, two in patients with chronic inflammatory disease and three tumor infiltrations. Youkey et al. (1983) also mentioned difficult dissections for retroperitoneal tumors as a special risk factor. Of 46 iatrogenic injuries reported by Pietri et al. (1981), one was an arterial lesion made during an extended hysterectomy. Especially in patients at increased risk of arteriosclerotic disease, the possibility of postoperative pelvic arterial occlusion with profound ischemia must be considered, one cause being retractor injury and another being damage during extensive intrapelvic dissection (Townsend et al. 1986).

Buri (1971) described a patient with profound bleeding during a cesarean section, where blind suture ligation of the right parametrium was undertaken. Four hours postoperatively, a relaparotomy was done and the hemorrhage was blamed on a coagulopathy. „Nur dem Mut und Einsatz der Anästhesistin war zu bedanken" that the patient was referred to a unit for vascular surgery where her lacerated external iliac artery and vein were repaired; the following course was uneventful.

In Table 3 are shown the Swedish cases identified in the questionnaire by Bergqvist and Bergqvist (1987). In all cases the predominating problem from the beginning was severe bleeding, the median peroperative blood loss being 11 l (range 0.7–15.1 l). This obviously indicates severe problems with hemostasis and perhaps also that the surgeon most competent to deal with bleeding complications was not at hand. Venous injuries dominated. In one patient the hemostatic procedure led to ligation of the external iliac artery and development of ischemia,

Table 3. Patients with vascular complications after laparotomy and vaginal operation. (After Bergqvist and Bergqvist 1987)

Patient no. Indication	Type of operation	Injured vessel	Symptoms	Management
1. Cancer colli uteri during pregnancy	Cesarean section + hysterectomy ad modum Wertheim	Right internal iliac vein	Bleeding	Suture ligation
2. Cancer colli uteri	Hysterectomy ad modum Wertheim	Inferior vena cava	Bleeding	Primary suture and then PTFE patch
3. Myoma	Hysterectomy + bilateral salpingo-oophorectomy	Right internal iliac vein	Bleeding	Suture ligation
4. Myoma	Hysterectomy + bilateral salpingo-oophorectomy	Right external iliac vein	Bleeding	Venorrhapy
5. Cancer corpus uteri (radiation)	Hysterectomy + bilateral salpingo-oophorectomy	Right external iliac artery	Peroperative bleeding + postoperative ischemia	Patch graft
6. Bilateral sactosalpinx	Bilateral salpingo-oophorectomy	Left external iliac vein	Peroperative bleeding + postoperative swelling	Saphenous graft × 2
7. Cervical	Hysterectomy ad modum Wertheim	Right internal iliac vein	Postoperative shock	Suture ligation
8. Myoma	Vaginal hysterectomy	Right internal iliac vein[a]	Postoperative bleeding	Suture ligation

[a] The ureter was damaged as well, necessitating reimplantation.

and in another ligation of the external iliac vein caused immediate and severe leg swelling.

There was no mortality, but there were quite a few complications and long-term sequelae. Patient 1 had profuse bleeding, and aortic compression was performed. The exact duration of compression was not recorded but it was certainly several minutes. Postoperatively, an electrocardiogram showed ischemic alterations. The two patients in whom vein reconstruction was performed (patients 2 and 6) were heparinized; both developed postoperative hematomas which had to be evacuated. Patient 3 was reoperated because of postoperative hypovolemia caused by hemorrhage from a prevesical artery. Patient 7 developed pneumothorax after insertion of a subclavian central venous catheter. Patient 4 had a wound infection and twice a cicatricial hernia. Thus, immediate postoperative complications were seen in six of the seven patients who underwent primary laparotomy. At follow-up 2 years later the patient with aortic compression (no. 1) had an S1 syndrome (i.e., neurological deficit corresponding to first sacral nerve damage). The two patients with vein reconstruction (nos. 2 and 6) had deep vein insufficiency after 1 year. In patient 2, venography revealed an occlusion of the left common iliac vein.

Delayed Problems

There have been 14 reported cases of development of arteriovenous fistulas (Antebi et al. 1974; Camp 1953; Decker et al. 1968; Elkin and Banner 1946; Field et al. 1963; Gaylis et al. 1973; Howard 1968; Swenson et al. 1978; Weed et al. 1975; Wideman 1979). The median time between the gynecologic operation and laparotomy for fistula was long – 8 years, with a range of 2 months to 21 years. The primary operations were hysterectomy in eight cases, in three of them combined with salpingo-oophorectomy, cesarean section in three cases, and myomectomy, unilateral salpingo-oophorectomy, and colporrhaphy in one case each. In only one patient was there a high-output cardiac failure (Camp 1953). The other patients had various more or less atypical symptoms (Table 4). The feeding artery was the uterine in seven cases, the ovarian in four cases, and the inferior vesical, common iliac, and pudendal in one case each. A typical finding was extensive venous dilatation with an aneurysmal appearance. In most of the cases the entire arteriovenous plexus was removed with good final results. In the patient with a

Table 4. Symptoms of arteriovenous fistula after gynecologic surgery in 14 cases reported in the literature

	No. of patients
Abdominal pain	7
Hip pain	3
Finding on palpation	4
Rectal perineal pain	1
Dyspareunia	1

fistula from the left common iliac artery ligation was tried, but the patient bled to death (Decker et al. 1968).

A special problem is encountered in patients with vulvar squamous cell carcinoma, where treatment involves radical vulvectomy and groin and pelvic lymphadenectomy. Especially when radiation treatment is given as well, there may be development of necrosis in the groin. As this area is easily infected, the necrosis can be florid and lead to involvement of the vessels, resulting in acute and severe hemorrhage (Deppe et al. 1984; Fuller 1979). Another situation in which massive vaginal hemorrhage may occur is during continuous cytostatic infusion in cases of recurrent or metastatic carcinoma of the cervix invading major vessels (Fuller 1979).

Prevention and Treatment

Major vascular injury during laparoscopy, although rare, is a real threat to the patient, and Corson (1980) states that these injuries are always due to operator error. It seems reasonable to accept a certain frequency of injuries, but they must be handled lege artis and the high mortality reported above is not acceptable. There are several moments during the laparoscopic procedure when injuries can be inflicted:
1. On insertion of the pneumoperitoneum needle.
2. On insufflation of the peritoneum.
3. On insertion of the trocar.
4. On insertion of the lateral accessory trocar.
5. During use of the biopsy forceps.
6. During electrocoagulation.

Prevention must be aimed at, and several points are worth mentioning.

First, the laparoscopic technique is important (Fig. 3). This has been discussed in detail by Penfield (1977). Injuries caused by the insufflation needle are just as common as injuries caused by the trocar. An off-center insertion of the instruments is recommended. Grasping the abdominal fascia and elevating it while the insufflation needle is inserted is very important, as is an adequate pneumoperitoneum, producing a very hard abdominal wall. The importance of experience and training has been illustrated by Mintz (1977). He surveyed 99 204 laparoscopies and found that the numbers of deaths, cardiorespiratory accidents, and laparotomies were significantly greater among beginners or teaching teams than among trained laparoscopists (> 800 laparoscopies). Especially in patients who have previously undergone laparotomy, the method described by Grundsell and Larsson (1982) should be considered. After incision of the skin and fascia, the peritoneum is penetrated by the index finger. A sharpened trocar is important. The patient should be in Trendelenburg's position.

Second, anatomic knowledge is important (Twombley 1973). Failure to note anatomic landmarks can lead to laparoscopic injury. The dominance of right-sided over left-sided iliac injuries is understandable, based on the anatomic location of the arteries.

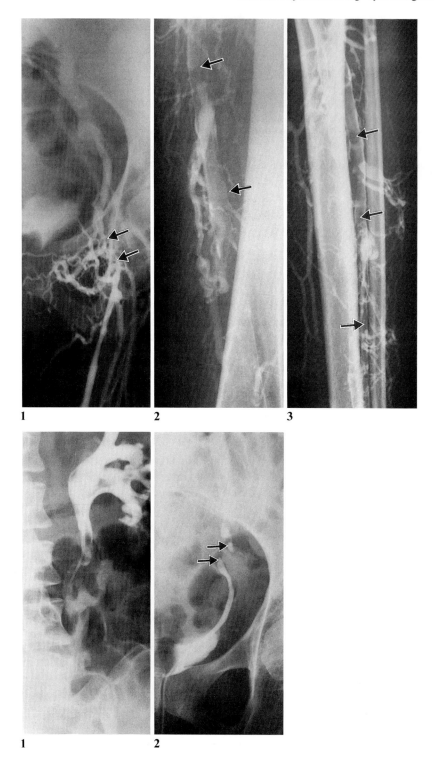

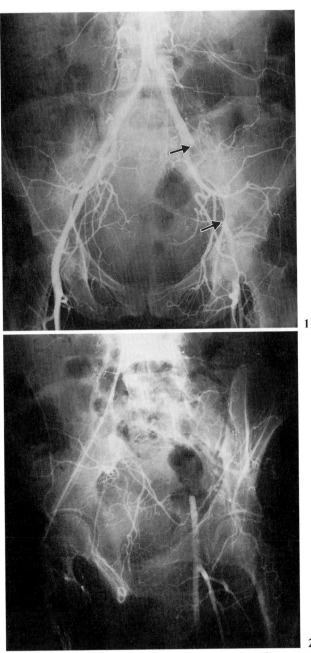

Fig. 2. Bleeding after laparoscopy. During surgery there were difficulties in localizing the source of bleeding and a hysterectomy was performed. Several suture ligations were made and postoperatively the patient developed a swollen leg, flank pain, and moderate ischemia. **a 1, 2, 3** Phlebograms showing the ligated femoral vein (*between arrows* in 1) with extensive thrombosis (*arrows*). **b 1, 2** The ligated ureter (*between arrows*) with hydronephrosis. **b 1** is an antegrade and **b 2** is a retrograde view. **c 1** The ligated iliac artery with occlusion (*arrows*) but a rich collateral network. **c 2** Filling of the normal common femoral artery

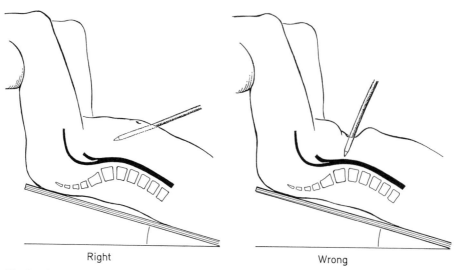

Right   Wrong

Fig. 3. The close relationship between the abdominal wall and the aorta means that adequate intra-abdominal insufflation and correct direction of the instruments are important during laparoscopy

Third, when there is a massive hemorrhage, blind attempts to achieve hemostasis worsen the situation in most cases. Gentle pressure is enough, and the problem should then be solved by a competent surgeon.

Fourth, especially in cases of laparoscopy, shock during or after the operation must always be considered as being hypovolemic until proven otherwise. Profuse bleeding during laparoscopy or shock afterwards indicates a necessity for laparotomy.

In cases of hemorrhage, both after laparoscopy and during laparotomy, it is extremely important to obtain adequate exposure of the bleeding site. This is the only way to make the hemostatic procedure adequate and safe and to obtain conditions for an optimal reconstruction. Ligation of both internal iliac arteries is sometimes recommended in desperate situations (e.g., see Reich and Nechtow 1961), but the rich collateral network sometimes prevents adequate hemostasis.

A special problem is met in patients in whom radical vulvectomy has been performed, especially when combined with groin lymphadenectomy and radiation therapy. Covering the vessels is important, and the possibility of transposing the sartorius muscle over the femoral triangle should be considered (Fuller 1979). In cases of vascular injury extra-anatomic reconstruction such as an obturator bypass is probably the method of choice (for further discussion, see chapter on radiation injuries).

The pathogenesis of arteriovenous fistulas is not fully known, but mass ligation, especially suture ligation of artery and vein, is probably one important mechanism. One way to prevent this, therefore, is to ligate artery and vein separately. There are two characteristics of arteriovenous fistulas after gynecological surgery. First, most of them are small and only rarely do they seem to induce heart failure. Second, all of them are associated with expanding venous aneurysms with very thin walls, and often with a venous plexus. This makes simple ligation difficult, and the treatment of choice should be total removal of the fistulous system, which often means hysterectomy and/or oophorectomy at the same time.

References

Antebi E, Adar R, Deutsch V, Mozes M (1974) Arteriovenous fistula complicating gynecologic operations. Obstet Gynecol 44:856–861
Bartsich EG, Dillon TF (1981) Injury of superior mesenteric vein. NY State J Med 81:933
Bergan J (1987) Litigation after acute vascular emergencies. In: Bergan J, Yao J (eds) Vascular surgical emergencies. Grune and Stratton, New York
Bergqvist D, Bergqvist A (1987) Vascular injuries during gynecologic surgery. Acta Obstet Gynecol Scand 66:19–23
Bistler H, Sinde J, Alemany J (1986) Verletzungen der großen Gefäße bei gynäkologischen Laparoskopien. Geburtshilfe Frauenheilkd 40:553–556
Boontje H (1981) Iatrogenic vascular trauma. Vasc Surg 15:266–271
Buri P (1971) Iatrogene Schädigung von Blutgefäßen. Helv Chir Acta 38:151–155
Buytaert P, Meulyzer P (1977) Gynecologic laparoscopy: a risk-free intervention? (in Dutch). Ned Tijdschr Geneeskd 121:397–401
Camp OB (1953) Arteriovenous fistula following hysterectomy. Am J Surg 86:240–243
Chapin JW, Hurlberg BJ, Scheer K (1980) Hemorrhage and cardiac arrest during laparoscopic tubal ligation. Anesthesiology 53:342–343
Cohen M (1971) Hazards of laparoscopy. Ariz Med 28:830
Corson SL (1980) Major vessel injury during laparoscopy. Am J Obstet Gynecol 138:589–590
Corson SL, Bolognese RJ (1972) Laparoscopy: an overview and results of a large series. J Reprod Med 9:148–157
Courey NG, Cunanan RG, Taefi O (1973) Sterilization via laparoscope. NY State J Med 73:559–561
DeBoer CH, Hutchins CJ (1975) Correspondence. Br Med J 2:137
Decker DG, Fish CR, Juergens JL (1968) Arteriovenous fistulas of the female pelvis. Obstet Gynecol 31:799–805
Deppe G, Malviya V, Smith P, Zbella E, Pildes R (1984) Limb salvage in recurrent vulvar carcinoma after rupture of femoral artery. Gynecol Oncol 19:120–124
Duignan NM, Jordan JA, Coughlan BM (1972) One thousand consecutive cases of diagnostic laparoscopy. J Obstet Gynecol Br Commonwealth 79:1016–1024
Elkin DC, Banner EA (1946) Arteriovenous aneurysm following surgical operations. JAMA 131:1117–1119
Erkrath KD, Weiler G, Adebahr G (1979) Zur Aortenverletzung bei Laparoskopie in der Gynäkologie. Geburtshilfe Frauenheilkd 79:687–689
Esposito JM (1973) Hematoma of the sigmoid colon as a complication of laparoscopy. Am J Obstet Gynecol 117:581–582
Esposito JM, Rubino G (1974) Bleeding after ovarian biopsy under laparoscopic vision. Am J Obstet Gynecol 119:857–858
Fear RE (1968) Laparoscopy: a valuable aid in gynecologic diagnosis. Obstet Gynecol 31:297–309
Field C, Welch J, Johnson C (1963) Posthysterectomy arteriovenous fistula involving uterine artery and vein. Am J Obstet Gynec 87:105–108
Frangenheim H (1971) Sicherheitsmaßnahmen zur Verhütung von Komplikationen bei der Laparoskopie. Endoscopy 3:10–20
Frenkel Y, Oelsner G, Ben-Baruch G, Menczer J (1981) Major surgical complications of laparoscopy. Eur J Obstet Gynecol Reprod Biol 12:107–111
Fuller A (1979) Life-threatening complications in the gynecologic cancer patient. Curr Probl Cancer 4:30–35

Gaylis H, Levine E, van Dongen LGR, Katz I (1973) Arteriovenous fistulas after gyneco-
  logic operations. Surg Gynecol Obstet 137:655–658
Grundsell H, Larsson G (1982) A modified laparoscopic entry technique using a finger.
  Obstet Gynecol 59:509–510
Havemann O, Kolmozen K, Hausswald H-R, Wergien G (1977) Komplikationen bei der
  gynäkologischen Laparoskopie. Zentralbl Gynakol 99:1186–1189
Heinrich P, Jahn R, Neumann A (1985) Iatrogene Gefäßschäden im Beckenbereich. Zen-
  tralbl Gynakol 107:432–434
Howard LR (1968) Iatrogenic arteriovenous sinus of a uterine artery and vein. Obstet
  Gynecol 31:255–257
Hulka JF, Soderström RM, Corson SL, Brooks PG (1973) Complications Committee of
  the American Association of Gynecological Laparoscopists: First annual report. J Re-
  prod Med 10:301–306
Katz M, Beck P, Tancer ML (1979) Major vessel injury during laparoscopy: anatomy of
  two cases. Am J Obstet Gynecol 135:544–545
Kurzel RB, Edinger DD (1983) Injury to the great vessels: a hazard of transabdominal en-
  doscopy. South Med J 76:656–657
Lignitz E, Püschel K, Saukko P, Koops E, Mattig W (1985) Iatrogene Blutungskomplika-
  tionen bei gynäkologischen Laparoskopien – Bericht über zwei Fälle mit tödlichem
  Verlauf. Z Rechtsmed 95:297–306
Loffer FD, Pent D (1975) Indications, contraindications and complications of laparos-
  copy. Obstet Gynecol Surg 30:407–427
Lord JW, Stone PW, Cloutier WA, Breidenbach L (1958) Major blood vessel injury during
  elective surgery. Arch Surg 77:282–288
Lübke F (1977) Komplikationen bei Laparoskopien. Arch Gynekol 224:282–283
Lynn SC, Katz AR, Ross PJ (1982) Aortic perforation sustained at laparoscopy. J Reprod
  Med 27:217–219
McDonald PT, Rich NM, Collins GJ, Andersen CA, Kozloff L (1978) Vascular trauma
  secondary to diagnostic and therapeutic procedures: laparoscopy. Am J Surg 135:651–
  655
Mintz M (1977) Risks and prophylaxis in laparoscopy: a survey of 100 000 cases. J Reprod
  Med 1977; 18:269–272
Moldin P, Jacobson M (1984) Gynecologic laparoscopy in routine health care – a prospec-
  tive study (in Swedish). Lakartidningen 81:4045–4048
Nilsen PA, Jerve F (1976) Tubal sterilization. With special reference to electrocoagulation
  through the laparoscope. Acta Obstet Gynecol Scand 55:349–353
Parewijck W, Thiery M, Timperman J (1979) Serious complications of laparoscopy. Med
  Sci Law 19:199–201
Penfield AJ (1977) Trocar and needle injuries. In: Phillips JM (ed) Laparoscopy. Williams
  and Wilkins, Baltimore, pp 236–241
Peterson HB, Greenspan JR, Ory HW (1982) Death following puncture of the aorta during
  laparoscopic sterilization. Obstet Gynecol 59:133–134
Pietri P, Alagni G, Settembrini PG, Gabrielli F (1981) Iatrogenic vascular lesions. Int Surg
  66:213–216
Reich W, Nechtow M (1961) Ligation of the internal iliac (hypogastric) arteries: a life-sav-
  ing procedure for uncontrollable gynecologic and obstetric hemorrhage. J Inte Coll
  Surg 36:157–168
Rich N, Hobson R, Fedde W (1974) Vascular trauma secondary to diagnostic and thera-
  peutic procedures. Am J Surg 128:715–721
Rust M, von Buquoy F, Bonke S (1980) Retroperitoneale Gefäßverletzung bei gynäkolo-
  gischen Laparoskopien. Anästh Intensivther Notfallmed 15:356–359
Schneller E, Felshart K, Fischmann S, Schwartz U, Bruntsch KH (1982) Operative Kom-
  plikationen der laparoskopischen Tubensterilisation mit dem Bleier-Clip (prospective
  Studie). Geburtshilfe Frauenheilkd 42:379–384
Shin CS (1982) Vascular injury secondary to laparoscopy. NY State J Med 82:935–936
Sirinek K, Levine B (1985) Traumatic injury to the proximal superior mesenteric vessels.
  Surgery 98:831–835

Swenson W, Tolstedt G, Ramos P, Peters C (1978) Ovarian arteriovenous fistula. An unusual cause of abdominal pain. Obstet Gynecol 62 [Suppl]:635
Townsend P, Hutson D, Lorecchio J, Averette H (1986) Acute peripheral arterial occlusion
  associated with surgery for gynecologic cancer. Gynecol Oncol 15:108–114
Twombly GH (1973) Hemorrhage in gynecologic surgery. Clin Obstet Gynecol 16:135–
  161
Youkey JR, Claget GP, Rich NM et al. (1983) Vascular trauma secondary to diagnostic
  and therapeutic procedures: 1974 through 1982. Am J Surg 146:788–791
Weed J, Hammond C, Clement E, McConnell R (1975) Ovarian arteriovenous fistula. Am
  J Obstet Gynecol 121:569–70
Wideman GL, Gravlee LC, Jones WN (1959) Arteriovenous aneurysm of the uterine artery
  and vein following total abdominal hysterectomy. Am J Obstet Gynecol 78:200–203

Injuries Caused by Diagnostic
and Therapeutic Interventions in Kidney and Urinary Tract

Types of Injury

Arteriovenous, extrarenal, or intrarenal fistulae, stenoses or occlusions of the renal artery or its branches, and extrarenal vascular lesions, including pelvic artery lesions following kidney transplantation, can be caused by diagnostic or therapeutic interventions.

Causes of Injury

Extrarenal arteriovenous fistulae are usually caused by nephrectomy with a mass ligature and transfixion suture of arteries and veins in the renal pedicle (Aravanis et al. 1962; Ditchek et al. 1969; Elkin 1948, 1971; Esquivel and Grabstald 1964; Gitlitz et al. 1963; Gokarn and Swinney 1962; Hollingsworth 1934; Papadopoulos and Manoli 1967; Shirey 1959), often combined with infection (Schwartz et al. 1955) or packing of the wound (Elliot 1961). A few cases of such fistulae have been caused by needle biopsy, during which the extrarenal artery and vein (Papadopoulos and Manoli 1967), or the subcostal vessels (Beisel et al. 1962; Fadhli and Derrick 1964; Slotkin and Madsen 1962) were perforated. An arteriovenous fistula has been a found between the renal artery and vein in a transplanted kidney (Pigott and Sharp 1987).

Intrarenal arteriovenous fistulae are usually due to needle biopsies (Bennett and Wiener 1965; Ekelund 1970; Elkin 1971; Kaufman et al. 1965; Kark et al. 1958; Moulonguet and Dufour 1970; Riley 1965; Sher 1969; Slotkin and Madsen 1962; Turner and Jacobsen 1965). It has been suggested that the kidney is particularly susceptible to fistulization because of the anatomic juxtaposition of the arcuate and interlobar arteries and veins, as well as the high blood flow through these vessels (Kaufman et al. 1965). Special factors, such as periarteritis nodosa (Curran et al. 1967), nephrosclerosis (Boijsen and Köhler 1962), and hypertension (Kark et al. 1958), have been suggested to increase the risk of this complication. Intrarenal arteriovenous fistulae have also been described after nephrolithotomy (Eriksson and Berglund 1974) and after partial nephrectomy (Elliot 1961; Houtappel and Reijns 1963).

Stenoses or occlusions of the renal artery or its branches have been described after renal surgery, particularly surgery of the renal pelvis, and after adrenal surgery (Andersson 1976; Andersson et al. 1979; Young et al. 1969). Such complications may also occur after selective renal artery catheterization for angiography (Bergentz et al. 1973; Gewertz et al. 1977; see also p. 8).

Extrarenal vascular lesions, resulting in massive hemorrhage, occur occasionally after renal transplantation. They are caused by deep wound infection or urinary leakage, leading to disrupture and hemorrhage from the anastomosis between the iliac artery and the renal artery (Blohmé and Brynger 1985; Nissen et al. 1975; Vidne et al. 1976). Ocassionally, a pseudoaneurysm may rupture months or even years after the initial procedure (Vidne et al. 1976). Damage to the external iliac artery has been reported following electrocoagulation of the ureter (Aboulker 1976; Piger and Maurer 1974). Damage to the external iliac and hypogastric arteries has been described after surgery of the ureter and bladder (Aboulker 1976).

Incidence

The incidence of *intrarenal arteriovenous fistulae* following needle biopsy is high. Bennett and Wiener (1965) performed renal angiography following 58 renal biopsies and found arteriovenous fistulae in 11 cases. Ekelund and Lindholm (1971) performed renal angiography between 3 and 1368 days after needle biopsy in 48 cases and found seven patients with arteriovenous fistulae. Since fistulae are mostly asymptomatic (Muth 1965) and are known to close spontaneously, the incidence may actually be higher in the early course after the biopsy. This assumption is supported by the results of immediately postoperative angiographic studies in 18 patients (Meng and Elkin 1971). In six of these minimal to extensive local accumulation of contrast medium was seen, as were minimal arteriovenous communication and nephrographic defects. In an experimental study in rabbits Ekelund demonstrated arteriovenous fistulae in not less than 16 of 36 animals 2 weeks after renal biopsies (Ekelund 1971).

Intrarenal arteriovenous fistulae may occur after needle biopsies of transplanted kidneys, but the incidence is unknown (Diaz-Buxo et al. 1974). The incidence of intrarenal arteriovenous fistulae for other reasons, as well as that of extrarenal arteriovenous fistulae, is low, and no series of such cases has been presented. The same is true for renal artery lesions caused by selective angiography and by renal surgery.

Blohmé and Brynger (1985) reported an incidence of arterial disrupture caused by septic arteritis following renal transplantation of 5.8% in their first 275 renal transplants (1965–1970). In their latest 459 transplants (1980–1984) the incidence had dropped to 0.4%.

Symptoms and Signs

Extrarenal arteriovenous fistulae are often large, causing general hemodynamic symptoms with cardiac insufficiency (Harbison et al. 1960; Maldonado et al. 1964; Sheps and Maldonado 1969; Shirey 1959). It often takes a long time, sometimes as long as 35 years, until the fistula is diagnosed (Aravanis et al. 1962; Gitlitz et al. 1963; Gokarn and Swinney 1962; McCutchean and Hara 1967; Muller

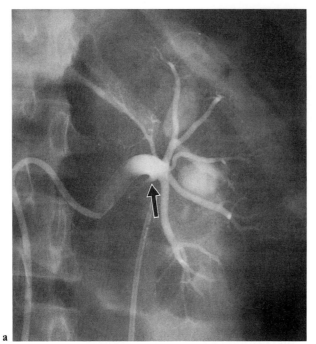

a

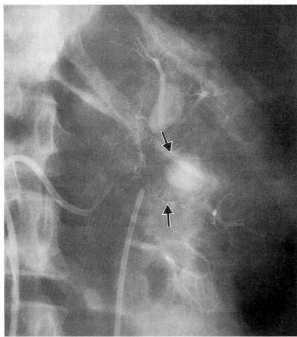

b

Fig. 1 a, b. A 21-year-old female patient had been operated on 6 months earlier because of pelvic staghorn calculus. During the operation the dorsal artery was damaged. After that operation she developed severe hypertension, angiography showing occlusion of the dorsal artery (**a** *arrow*) and a rich collateral network (**b** *arrows*). There is a urinary catheter with the tip in the renal pelvis. (Courtesy of Dr. Sverker Hellsten, Department of Urology, General Hospital, Malmö, Sweden)

and Goodwin 1956). A flank bruit is an important diagnostic sign. The shunting of blood causes some degree of renal ischemia, which may result in hypertension and, if the kidney function is impaired, in a rise in serum creatinine (Moulonguet and Dufour 1970). Occasionally, however, there is a lowering of the blood pressure due to cardiac insufficiency, which is normalized after operative treatment (Brandt 1963).

Intrarenal arteriovenous fistulae are usually small and asymptomatic. Hematuria has been described (Moulonguet and Dufour 1970; Fernström and Lindblom 1962). They have rarely been found to cause general hemodynamic disturbances, but a bruit is often heard over the kidney. They do cause a local redistribution of the blood flow, however, resulting in decreasing flow to the renal parenchyma with a tendency to hypertension (Smith et al. 1968) and impaired function of the affected kidney (Lingårdh et al. 1971). This mechanism has been studied by Lindgårdh et al. (1971) using the dye-dilution technique. Small fistula are visualized by the injection of angiotensin (Ekelund et al. 1972).

Stenotic or occlusive lesions of the renal artery or its branches may cause infarction of the kidney or part of the kidney, or an ischemic area resulting in hypertension (Fig. 1) and, more rarely, uremia (Bergentz et al. 1973).

Anastomotic disrupture after renal transplantation results in massive hemorrhage, which sometimes is fatal. When a pseudoaneurysm is formed it is often large and can be felt as a pulsating tumor (Blohmé and Brynger 1985; Nissen et al. 1975; Vidne et al. 1976).

Prophylactic Measures

In studies on rabbits, Ekelund demonstrated that premedication with an antifibrinolytic agent (tranexamic acid) markedly decreased the number of arteriovenous fistulae following renal biopsy (Ekelund 1972). No clinical studies have been reported.

Careful anatomic dissection, avoiding mass ligation, will probably decrease the incidence of postoperative arteriovenous fistulae.

Management of the Lesions

Extrarenal arteriovenous fistulae must often be operated on. This is done by dissection and isolation of the renal artery and vein and individual ligation of these structures, if the kidney has been removed, which usually is the case. Otherwise the fistulous tract has to be isolated and divided. Even major extrarenal arteriovenous fistulae may close spontaneously (Halpern 1969).

Intrarenal arteriovenous fistulae have a strong tendency to spontaneous closure. Bennett and Wiener (1965) followed such fistulae angiographically in six patients and found that three had disappeared, one had decreased, and two persisted. Nilsson and Ross (1969) described closure of both bilateral arteriovenous fistulae in one patient, and Ekelund and Lindholm (1971) closure of the fistulae in five of seven patients, all studied with repeated arteriography after 1 or a few

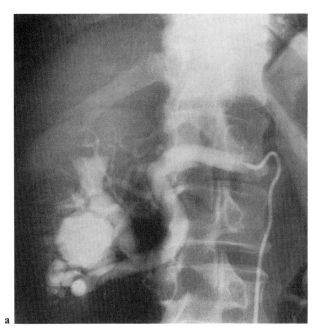

a

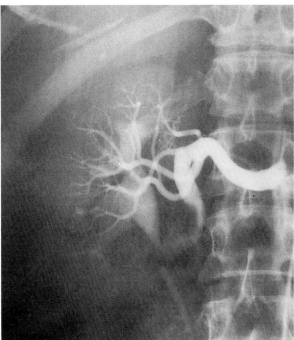

b

Fig. 2a, b. A 51-year-old male patient was evaluated because of renovascular hypertension. A significant left-sided renal artery stenosis was detected and at the same time an intrarenal arteriovenous fistula was seen in the right kidney (**a**) where a needle biopsy had been made 13 years previously. The renal artery stenosis was corrected with a patch angioplasty and on the follow-up angiogram 1 week later there were no signs of the arteriovenous fistula (**b**). The loud bruit heard before surgery had disappeared

years. Experimentally, Ekelund (1971) studied 20 rabbits with arteriovenous fistulae and demonstrated closure in 14 (70%) in 3 months, decrease in size in three and persistence in three. It is therefore obvious that there is a strong tendency of these fistulae to closure, but this sometimes takes a long time.

We recently experienced the spontaneous closure of an asymptomatic fistula following needle biopsy after 13 years (Fig. 2 a). The closure occurred after the patient had been operated on for renovascular hypertension, caused by a stenosis on the *contralateral* renal artery. The operation was successful and resulted in a decrease of the blood pressure. The closure of the fistula, which occurred a few days after surgery, was demonstrated by the disappearance of a bruit and was confirmed angiographically (Fig. 2b). The spontaneous closure of the fistula was most probably due to a combination of a lowered blood pressure after reconstruction of the contralateral artery stenosis and the hypercoagulable state induced by surgery.

Operative closure of intrarenal arteriovenous fistulae has been reported, particularly of fistulae occurring after nephrolithotomy (Eriksson and Berglund 1974) and after partial nephrectomy (Boijsen and Köhler 1962). Such a procedure requires dissection of each renal artery and vein as well as of the vessels feeding and draining the fistula. These vessels have to be identified and ligated separately (Kaufman et al. 1965). Due to technical difficulties, nephrectomy has been performed in some cases of intrarenal fistulae (Snodgrass and Robinson 1964).

Since intrarenal arteriovenous fistulae have a strong tendency to spontaneous closure and are rarely symptomatic, operative intervention is not often indicated (Curran et al. 1967; Halpern 1969).

Occlusions or stenoses of the renal artery or one of its branches may require surgical therapy due to severe hypertension and/or impaired kidney function. Gewertz et al. (1977) reported four cases of intraluminal catheter-induced intima dissections of the renal artery, causing renovascular hypertension. One case was treated with an aortorenal saphenous vein graft and two with nephrectomy, while the fourth did not require treatment. Bergentz et al. (1973) reported a case of severe hypertension following catheter-induced occlusion of a supplemental renal artery, treated with ex-vivo reconstruction and autotransplantation.

Andersson et al. (1979) describe two cases of hypertension following renal artery branch ligation in connection with pyelolithotomy, requiring nephrectomy. Persistent hypertension after surgery for pheochromocytoma may be due to accidental ligation of a renal artery branch and may necessitate nephrectomy (Young et al. 1969).

Hemorrhage from an iliac artery-renal artery anastomosis in kidney transplantation requires immediate exploration. Since the bleeding is practically always caused by a septic process, the leakage should not be resutured, but the artery ligated and the transplanted kidney removed. If the anastomosis was performed between the external iliac artery and the renal artery, ligation of the former artery is necessary. If the anastomosis was performed between the hypogastric artery and the renal artery, ligation of the hypogastric artery is usually sufficient. Due to spread of the infection, ligation of the common iliac artery may be necessary, however. Ligation of the external or common iliac artery can usually be performed in these patients without serious sequelae, as reported by Gorey et al. (1979) and by Blohmé and Brynger (1985). If severe ischemia develops a femorofemoral bypass can be performed. However, there is a risk of spreading the infection, either directly, due to the proximity of the infected area, or due to bacteremia. Simple ligation may therefore be the procedure of choice in the acute stage, followed by careful clinical observation of the patient.

References

Aboulker P (1976) Les lésions artérielles au cours de la chirurgie urinaire. Ann Urol (Paris) 10:1–3

Andersson I (1976) Renal artery lesions after pyelolithotomy. A potential cause of renovascular hypertension. Acta Radiol Diagn 17:685–695

Andersson I, Boijsen E, Hellsten S, Linell F (1979) Lesions of the dorsal renal artery in surgery for renal pelvic calculus. Eur Urol 5:343–346

Aravanis C, Michaelides G, Alivizatos CN, Lazarides D (1962) Renal arterio-venous fistula following nephrectomy. Ann Surg 156:749–751

Beisel WR, Scalettar R, Barry KG (1962) Delayed vascular complications of renal biopsy. Med Ann 31:626–629

Bennett AR, Wiener SN (1965) Intrarenal arteriovenous fistula and aneurysm. A complication of percutaneous renal biopsy. AJR 95:372–382

Bennett WM, Strong D, Rosch J (1976) Arteriovenous fistula complicating renal transplantation. Urology 8:254

Bergentz S-E, Faarup P, Hegedüs V, Lindholm T, Lindstedt E (1973) Diagnosis of hypertension due to occlusion of a supplemental renal artery; its localization, treatment by removal from the body, microsurgical repair and reimplantation: a case report. Ann Surg 178:643–647

Blohmé I, Brynger H (1985) Emergency ligation of the external iliac artery. Ann Surg 201:505–510.

Boijsen E, Köhler R (1962) Renal arteriovenous fistulae. Acta Radiol 57:433–445

Brandt JL: (1963) Hypertension following closure of a postnephrectomy arteriovenous fistula: a case report and hypothesis. Can Med Assoc J 89:405–409

Curran RE, Steinberg I, Hagström JWC (1967) Arteriovenous fistula complicating percutaneous renal biopsy in polyarteritis nodosa. Am J Med 43:465–470

Diaz-Buxo JA, Kopen DF, Donadio JV (1974) Renal allograft arteriovenous fistula following percutaneous biopsy. J Urol 112:577–580

Ditchek T, Newman H, Diserens R, Harris K (1969) Arteriovenous fistula of renal vessels. J Urol 101:653–655

Ekelund L (1970) Arteriovenous fistulae secondary to renal biopsy. Acta Radiol [Diagn] (Stockh) 10:218–224

Ekelund L (1971) Spontaneous closure of arteriovenous fistulae following percutaneous renal biopsy. An experimental investigation in the rabbit. Acta Radiol [Diagn] (Stockh) 11:289–294

Ekelund L (1972) Prevention of arteriovenous fistula following renal biopsy by antifibrinolytic premedication. Scand J Urol Nephrol 6:81–83

Ekelund L, Göthlin J, Olin T (1972) Arteriovenous fistulae in rabbit kidney studied by dye-dilution technique and by angiography. Scand J Urol Nephrol 6:84–90

Ekelund L, Lindholm T (1971) Arteriovenous fistulae following percutaneous renal biopsy. Acta Radiol [Diagn] (Stockh) 11:38–48

Elkin D (1948) Aneurysm following surgical procedures. Ann Surg 127:769–779

Elkin M (1971) Renal vascular shunts. Clin Radiol 22:156–170

Elliot JA (1961) Post-nephrectomy arteriovenous fistula. J Urol 85:426–427

Eriksson I, Berglund G (1974) Intrarenal arteriovenous fistula after nephrolithotomy. Scand J Urol Nephrol 8:73–76

Esquivel EL, Grabstald H (1964) Renal arteriovenous fistula following nephrectomy for renal cell cancer. J Urol 92:367–376

Fadhli HA, Derrick JR (1964) Arteriovenous fistula – a complication of needle renal biopsy; case report and review of the literature. Am Surg 30:654–655

Fernström I, Lindblom K (1962) Selective renal biopsy using roentgen television control. J Urol 88:709–712

Gewertz BL, Stanley JC, Fry WJ (1977) Renal artery dissections. Arch Surg 122:409–414

Gitlitz GF, Fell SC, Sagerman RH, Hurwitt ES (963) Postnephrectomy arteriovenous fistula: case report and review of literature. Ann Surg 157:511–515

Gokarn A, Swinney J (1962) Arteriovenous aneurysm of the renal artery after nephrectomy. Br J Urol 34:15–18

Gorey TF, Bulkley GB, Spees EK, Sterioff S (1979) The relative paucity of ischemic sequelae in renal transplant patients. Ann Surg 190:756

Halpern M (1969) Spontaneous closure of traumatic renal arteriovenous fistulas. AJR 107:730–736

Harbison SP, Gregg FJ, Gutierrez IZ (1960) Arteriovenous fistula following nephrectomy: report of a case complicated by severe azotemia and congestive failure. Ann Surg 152:281–283

Hollingsworth EW (1934) Arteriovenous fistula of the renal vessels. Am J Med Sci 188:399–403

Houtappel HCEM, Reijns GA (1963) Intrahilar arteriovenous fistula following lower pole resection of the kidney. A case report and a review of the literature. Arch Chir Neer 15:45–65

Kark RM, Muehrcke RC, Pollak VE, Pirani CL, Kiefer JH (1958) An analysis of five hundred percutaneous renal biopsies. Arch Intern Med 101:439–451

Kaufman JJ, Gordon A, Maxwell MH (1965) Intrarenal arteriovenous fistula following needle biopsy of the kidney. Calif Med 103:350–354

Lingårdh G, Lindqvist B, Lundström B (1971) Renal arteriovenous fistula following puncture biopsy. A hemodynamic and functional study in four cases. Scand J Urol Nephrol 5:181–189

Maldonado JE, Sheps SG, Bernatz PE, DeWeerd JH, Harrison EG (1964) Renal arteriovenous fistula; a reversible cause of hypertension and heart failure. Am J Med 37:499

McCutcheon FB, Hara M (1967) Arteriovenous fistula following nephrectomy. J Cardiovasc Surg (Torino) 8:253–255

Meng C-H, Elkin M (1971) Immediate angiographic manifestations of iatrogenic renal injury due to percutaneous needle biopsy. Radiology 100:335–341

Moulonguet A, Dufour B (1970) Fistules artério-veineuses rénales traumatiques a propos d'un cas après biopsie „hépatique". J Urol Nephrol (Paris) 3:221–229

Muller WH, Goodwin WE (1956) Renal arteriovenous fistula following nephrectomy. Ann Surg 144:240–244

Muth RG (1965) The safety of percutaneous renal biopsy: an analysis of 500 consecutive cases. J Urol 94:1–3

Nilsson CG, Ross RJ (1969) Bilateral renal arteriovenous fistulas and decreased blood pressure following renal biopsies. J Urol 97:176–179

Nissen HM, Sorensen BL, Wolf H, Tonnesen KH (1975) Sudden massive hemorrhage after renal transplantation. Scand J Urol Nephrol 9:273–276

Papadopoulos CD, Manoli A (1967) Renal arteriovenous fistulae; review of the literature and report of a successfully treated case. Surgery 62:285–289

Piger A, Maurer P (1974) Zweiseitige Perforation der Arteria iliaca externa nach endoskopischer Ureterkoagulation. Med Monatsschr 28:310–311

Pigott JP, Sharp WV (1987) Arteriovenous fistula involving a transplant kidney. Transplantation 44:156–157

Riley JM (1965) Renal arteriovenous fistula: a complication of percutaneous renal biopsy. J Urol 93:333–335

Schwartz JW, Borski AA, Jahnke EJ (1955) Renal arteriovenous fistula. Surgery 37:951–954

Sheps SG, Maldonado JE (1969) Die arteriovenöse Nierenfistel. Ein Überblick über 109 Fälle. Klin Wochenschr 47:621–628

Sher MH (1969) Intrarenal arteriovenous fistula: a complication of needle biopsy. Am Surg 35:433–434

Shirey EK (1959) Cardiac disease secondary to postnephrectomy arteriovenous fistula. Report of a case. Cleve Clin Q 26:188–200

Slotkin EA, Madsen PO (1962) Complications of renal biopsy: incidence in 5000 reported cases. J Urol 87:13–15

Smith GH, Remmers AR, Dickey BM, Sarles HE (1968) Intrarenal arteriovenous fistula and systemic hypertension following percutaneous renal biopsy. Report of a case. Nephron 5:24–30

Snodgrass WT, Robinson MJ (1964) Intrarenal arteriovenous fistula: a complication of partial nephrectomy. J Urol 91:135–136

Turner AF, Jacobson G (1965) Renal arteriovenous fistulas following percutaneous renal biopsy. Radiology 85:460–461

Tyson KRT, Derrick JR. Renal arteriovenous fistula after nephrectomy: a case report. South Med J 55:558–560

Vidne BA, Leapman SB, Butt KM, Kountz SL (1976) Vascular complications in human renal transplantation. Surgery 79:77–81

Young TD, Quereski AS, Connor TB, Wiswell JG (1969) Problem lesions in adrenal surgery. J Urol 101:233

Iatrogenic Vascular Neck Injuries

Types of Injury

Tracheoarterial fistulas, arteriovenous fistulas, and hemorrhage due to vessel injury are possible complications of surgery in the neck area.

Very little is written about iatrogenic vascular injuries that occur during surgical procedures in the neck region in spite of the large and important vessels passing through the area. One reason is probably that surgeons operating in this region know how to handle intraoperative injuries and the lack of data in the literature is most likely a matter of underreporting. The predominating and most dramatic injury is tracheoarterial fistula in patients with tracheostomies. Injuries causing more long-term problems are arteriovenous fistulas, most frequently reported after thyroid surgery.

Arterial Injuries in Connection with Tracheostomy

Acute hemorrhage from an injured artery may occur during tracheostomy. These are sometimes due to anatomic variations of the aorta and the brachiocephalic trunk or to the presence of an arteria thyreoidea ima (Greenway 1972; Kia-Noury and Deubzer 1963; Potondi and Pribilla 1966). Laceration of the common carotid artery has also been reported during emergency tracheostomy (Lord et al. 1958). Early bleeding is seen within a few hours and depends on incomplete hemostasis, most frequently from isthmic or pretracheal veins or branches of the inferior laryngeal artery. In cases of vein injury, at least a theoretically possible complication is air embolization.

Late bleeding is seen within days or months and can be caused by (a) most often, an infectious hemorrhagic tracheobronchitis, (b) coagulation defects, (c) malignant tumors, or (d) tracheoarterial fistulae.

Tracheoarterial Fistulae

The first report of this complication was published in 1879, by Körte, and involved a patient with diphteria. Another patient, a small girl, was described by Frühwald in 1885, and in 1892 a series was published by Foltanek on hemorrhage after tracheotomy in patients with diphtheria, causing, among other things, arteriotracheal communications with heavy and lethal bleeding. The first reviews were written in 1900 by Engelhardt and in 1903 by Martina, and further review articles have been published since (Schlaepfer 1924; von Bihler and Hutschen-

Table 1. Incidence of tracheoarterial fistulas in connection with tracheostomy; only cases verified by autopsy have been registered

Reference	Period	No. of tracheostomies	No. of fistulas
Castaing et al. (1966)	1963–1966 Bordeaux	560	10
Adolfsson et al. (1975)	1965–1974 Umeå	1000	2
Arola et al. (1979)	1964–1975 Turku	816	5
Jones et al. (1976)	1964–1976 New Orleans	1501	10
Pfretzschner et al. (1973)	1958–1969 Munich	528	4
Mulder and Rubush (1969)	1963–1968 Iowa City	428	2
Rogers (1969)	1962–1965	549	3
Watts (1963)	1953–1960 Melbourne	212	0
Miech et al. (1967)	Strasbourg	229	3
Deslauriers et al. (1975)	Toronto	100	8
Arbulu and Thoms (1974)	1970–1973 Detroit	13	1
Vic-Dupont et al. (1967)	Paris	828	6
Grillo (1975)	Boston	139	1
Mounier-Kuhn et al. (1968)	Lyon	835	2
Rabuzzi et al. (1973)	1968–1972 Upstate N.Y.	23	1
De Montmollin (1962)	1955–1959 Zürich	625	5
Kantawala et al. (1972)	1970 Bombay	320	1
von Bihler and Hutschenreuter (1966)	1961–1965 Saar	182	1

reuter 1966; Mulder and Rubush 1969; Brantigan 1973; Lane et al. 1975; Jones et al. 1976). Though it was at first almost exclusively an injury that occurred in diphtheritic children, today other underlying diseases predominate, reflecting the altered indications for tracheostomy. Untreated, this complication has a 100% mortality, and even with treatment there are only a few long-term survivors.

The incidence of tracheoarterial fistulae is low (Table 1), but it is definitely higher in patients who have undergone tracheal resection because of tracheal stenosis, either with primary anastomosis or with some form of graft (Deslauriers et al. 1975; Arola et al. 1979; Arbula and Thoms 1974; Conrad et al. 1977; J. Donahoo, in Cooper 1977; Grillo 1975; Revilla et al. 1974; Weissman 1974). The frequency after ordinary tracheostomies varies between 0.3% and 1.8% (von Bihler and Hutschenreuter 1966), while it is 0.7%–8% after surgery for tracheal stenosis. Deslauriers et al. (1975) found four cases in which tracheal resection and end-to-end anastomosis had been done and four of seven cases when a Marlex prosthesis was used.

There are several predisposing factors which may be important for the development of a fistula:
1. Placement of the tracheostomy below the third tracheal ring (Brantigan 1973; Cooper 1977; Pusterla 1968; Thompson 1966)
2. Anatomic variations in the origin of the arteries from the aortic arch (McDonald and Anson 1940), with abberrant arteries (Selking et al. 1977; Jones et al. 1976), high crossing of the brachiocephalic trunk (Davis and Southwick 1956; Duval et al. 1969; von Strauchmann and Wagemann 1981),

or anteroposition of it (Gross and Withalm 1953; Couraud et al. 1967; Missionznik 1928). There are two cases known of tracheal fistula to a lusoric artery (Dotzauer and Althoff 1966; Miech et al. 1967). Lusoric artery (from *lusus naturae* = freak of nature) is the term for an anomalous right subclavian artery arising from the distal portion of the aortic arch, distal to the origin of the left subclavian artery. It crosses the midline between the spine and esophagus in 80% of cases, between the esophagus and trachea in 15%, and in front of both in 5%. The autopsy incidence is 0.4%–2% (for review, see Felson et al. 1950). Hewitt et al. (1970) have reviewed the most common types of aortic arch anomalies. Especially in children, the brachiocephalic trunk is often situated higher than expected (Kia-Noury and Deubzer 1963).

3. Thoracic deformity causing displacement of the aortic arch (Adolfson et al. 1975)
4. Exaggerated hyperextension of the head during the surgical procedure (Majeski and MacMillan 1978)
5. Excessively long or curved tracheal tube (von der Emde et al. 1976)
6. Frequent movements of the tube (Hood and Rush 1962): Donovan et al. (1977) reported on a patient with hemorrhage following multiple seizures; frequent coughing with movement between the tissues (Welin 1964); frequent manipulations with and changes of the tube (Castaing et al. 1966; Conn 1969)
7. Prolonged or high cuff or cannula pressure (Bertelsen and Jensen 1987; Lewis and Ranade 1978; Silén and Spieker 1965; Stiles 1965)
8. Infections in the trachea (Pathak 1969; Clin 1963; Biller and Ebert 1970; Subotié 1963; Myers et al. 1972; Jones et al. 1976; Brantigan 1973), *Pseudomonas aeruginosa* (or *P. pyocynea*) producing particularly large areas of erosion in a high frequency (Kmiecik et al. 1976; Neumann 1974)
9. Operation for tracheal stenosis (see above)
10. Defective nutritional status with negative nitrogen balance (Subotié 1963; Majeski and MacMillan 1978; Tilney and McArdle 1975; Jones et al. 1976; Majeski and MacMillan 1978)
11. Treatment with steroids (Vic-Dupont et al. 1967; Andrews and Pearson 1971; Jones et al. 1976; Majeski and MacMillan 1978; Selking et al. 1977)
12. Malignant process (Marcorelli 1968)

Since around 1950, 155 cases of tracheoarterial fistulas have been reported (67 male patients, 71 female patients, 17 patients of unreported gender). The median age was 24 (4–85) years and the predominating indication for tracheostomy was trauma (43 cases), followed by various infections (29), postoperative respiratory insufficiency (21), operation for tracheal stenosis (15), neurologic disorders (15), intoxication (13), and various other indications in the remaining 19 cases. The median time interval between tracheostomy and the large hemorrhage leading to death or operation was 8 days, with a range of 1 day to 21 months. Thus, in most cases the bleeding occurred in near temporal relationship to the tracheostomy, but there may be a considerable delay. In 20 cases the hemorrhage occurred more than a month after the tracheostomy (Adolfsson et al. 1975; Castaing et al. 1966; Davis and Southwick 1956; DeMontmollin 1962; Jones et al. 1976; Johnson 1951; Langlois et al. 1967; Lane et al. 1975; Lunding 1964; Majeski and MacMillan

1978; Mounier-Kuhn et al. 1968; Mehalic and Farhat 1972; Nunn et al. 1975; Reich and Rosenkrantz 1968; Toty et al. 1967; Vic-Dupont et al. 1967; Weissman 1974). In 63 cases there were one or more minor incidents of bleeding prior to the large one, in 27 cases there was a massive hemorrhage without warning, and in 27 cases there was no report of "herald" bleeding. Minor bleeding from the tracheostoma may be due to hemorrhagic tracheobronchitis, but when it occurs, a major artery erosion should nonetheless be suspected. In their review, Mulder and Rubush (1969) found 14 cases of bleeding among 428 cases of tracheostomy, 12 being due to tracheobronchitis and only two to a tracheoarterial fistula (to the innominate artery). In addition to herald bleeding, a pulsating tube is a warning sign (Davies and Southwick 1956). In 143 cases a fistula was situated between the trachea and the brachiocephalic trunk, in two cases to the inferior thyroid artery (Arola et al. 1979; Krejovic and Jorgacevic 1971), in four cases to the right common carotid artery (Kia-Noury and Deubzer 1963; DeMontmollin 1962), in one to the bifurcation of the brachiocephalic trunk into the subclavian and carotid arteries (Johnson 1951), in one to the right subclavian artery (Jones et al. 1976), in one to the left carotid artery (Schenken and Brown 1954), and in one to the thyreoidea ima branch from the brachiocephalic trunk (Willerson and Fred 1965). In two cases the fistula communicated with a lusoric artery (Dotzauer and Althoff 1966; Miech et al. 1967). Ninety cases were fatal and verified at autopsy, and in 64 cases an operation was undertaken. A total of 94 patients died of the hemorrhage, 13 died of other causes, mostly of complications to the trauma or disease because of which the tracheostomy had been performed, and in only 29 cases was there long-term survival.

The diagnosis may be difficult. Diagnostic angiography has been used, but it is often impossible to demonstrate the lesion in stable patients. In emergency situations there is seldom time for angiography (Conrad et al. 1977).

Table 2 shows the outcome in the patients who underwent emergency surgery. Although it is a relatively small group, it is evident that every form of primary reconstruction must be avoided because of the high frequency of rebleeding, often with a fatal outcome (Adolfsson et al. 1975; Bertelsen and Jensen 1987; Caterine

Table 2. Outcome of emergency surgery in patients with tracheoarterial fistula

Type of operation	No. of cases	No. of fatal cases	Mortality (%)
Suture ± patch graft	13	11	85
Vein bypass	9	4 ⎫	
Dacron bypass	3	1 ⎬	42
Resection + ligation or suture	33 [a, b]	3	9
Ligation + extraanatomic bypass	1	1	
Mors in tabula	5		

[a] In two patients (Jones et al. 1976) primary suture was done, in one case with a vein patch, but rebleeding occurred after 1 and 3 days respectively. After resection and ligation the patients survived.
[b] Two patients had long-term minor sequelae – mild left-sided neurologic deficit in one and right-sided arm claudication in the other.

1977; Comer et al. 1974; Elstein et al. 1971; Deslauriers et al. 1975; Jones et al. 1976; Lane et al. 1975; Myers et al. 1972; Prenner et al. 1972; Ramesh and Gazzaniga 1978; Selking et al. 1977; Silén and Spieker 1965). In one of the ligated cases new bleeding occurred after 4 days due to slipping of the distal ligature (Rydberg et al. 1972).

Prevention

Knowledge of the vascular anatomy is important, as is knowledge of anatomic variants. Scheldrup (1957) published an anatomic review to be used in cases of tracheotomy. The most common types of aortic arch anomalies have been reviewed by Hewitt et al. (1970) and McDonald and Anson (1940). One common variant is the passage of the right carotid and subclavian arteries in front of the trachea (Jarvis 1964; Pfretzschner et al. 1973; Courcy et al. 1985). Another, seen in 9% of the population, according to Potondi (1969), is the origin of the left common carotid artery from the brachiocephalic trunk.

When the neck is hyperextended during tracheostomy, the tracheal rings are moved upwards, causing the incision to be made lower than is realized (Ivankovic et al. 1969). A low tracheostomy places the tube closer to the brachiocephalic trunk (Cooper 1971; Brantigan 1973; Lane et al. 1975). The tracheostomy is preferably performed at the second or third tracheal ring.

Rigid tubes made of stainless steal or silver have a greater tendency to erode the tissue than do plastic or rubber ones (Mathog et al. 1971; Nunn et al. 1975). If the tube bend is 90° and the tracheostomy low, the inner "elbow" of the tube tends to erode the artery immediately below the stoma. This is especially the case if the tube is loaded with absorbers. An angle of 60° is preferred (Utley et al. 1972). Frequent movements of a poorly fitting tube may cause erosion by the tip. The cuff pressure should be less than 25 mm Hg to avoid pressure necrosis (Ching et al. 1974). Low-pressure cuffs are thus important in reducing tracheal damage (Grillo et al. 1971; Weiss et al. 1976). In dogs it has been shown that a small air leakage passing the cuff gives a lower frequency of tracheal erosions than is obtained with various patterns for intermittent cuff deflation (Bryant et al. 1971). Totally incorrect placing of the tube outside the trachea may cause vascular necrosis (Veress and Romhanyi 1965). Erosion is accelerated by infection (Arola et al. 1979), and prophylaxis against infection must therefore be rigorous. Great care must be taken when changing tubes and when suctioning. To avoid unnecessary movements, cough suppression is important. Decannulation or a change of cannula are dangerous moments, requiring increased patient observation (Mayer 1957).

As surgery for tracheal stenosis is an important risk factor, it has been recommended that some tissue be interposed between the artery and the tracheal anastomosis, e.g., a pericardial buttress (Arbulu and Thoms 1974), the superior pole or upper body of the thymus gland, or a pedicle of the sternothyroid (Deslauriers et al. 1975) or sternocleidomastoid muscles (Castaing et al. 1966). If muscle interposition is used the muscular tissue must be adequately vascularized (von Moritz 1978).

Diagnosis

In cases with herald bleeding or a pulsating tracheal tube, where the presence of a gross arterial erosion must be suspected, very little help has been obtained by various diagnostic modalities. Jones et al. (1976) analyzed various diagnostic attempts such as bronchoscopy, aortic arch angiography, retrograde brachial arteriography, and surgical exploration of the wound. Only rarely was the correct diagnosis obtained, and in may cases with profound bleeding there is no time to perform various diagnostic maneuvers, particularly angiography.

Treatment

As tracheoarterial bleeding is highly lethal and, moreover, rare, there must be a well-formulated plan of management in case the complication occurs. Jones et al. (1976) concluded that all patients having lost over 10 ml of blood from the tracheostoma or cannula more than 48 h after the tracheostomy must be assumed to have a tracheoarterial fistula until proven otherwise. Careful examination should be done in the operating room. After balloon deflation and decannulation, inspection of the trachea should be done with a fiberoptic bronchoscope. Blood clots should be carefully removed, and if significant bleeding occurs cuff inflation is done, followed by a median sternotomy.

The development of massive bleeding from a patient's tracheostomy is a surgical emergency. Preliminary hemostasis should first be tried by cuff inflation if the cuff has been deflated. It is also important at this moment to secure a free airway. According to Brantigan (1973), balloon tamponade was successful in 17 of 23 cases and, according to Jones et al. (1976), in 28 of 34 cases. Gauze has also been recommended (Myers and Pilch 1969), but care must be taken to garantee a free airway. Endotracheal tube insertion is successful in about one third of the cases (Jones et al. 1976). If the measures mentioned above do not stop the bleeding, blunt finger dissection behind the sternum and digital compression of the brachiocephalic trunk against the sternum are almost always enough to obtain hemostasis (Fig. 1; Utley et al. 1972; Fox 1973; Jones et al. 1976; Caterine 1977). The patient must be taken to the operating room immediately. The arteries are approached via a median sternotomy, and it is possible to prolong the incision in the right side of the neck. Resection of the left innominate vein is usually not necessary, except when it is involved in the necrotic tissue (Cooper 1977). Prenner et al. (1972) recommended primary suture of the defect but, as discussed above, this must be rejected because of the great risk of new arterial necrosis with fatal rebleeding. The method of choice is resection of the eroded artery and ligation or suture of the arterial stumps after adequate débridement. In cases of fistula to the brachiocephalic artery, which by far predominate, the aim must be to maintain communication between the carotid and subclavian arteries. Sutures must be placed in a healthy arterial wall and monofilament suture material should be used.

In the majority of people it is possible to divide the innominate artery without producing contralateral neurologic defects or ischemic symptoms in the ipsilat-

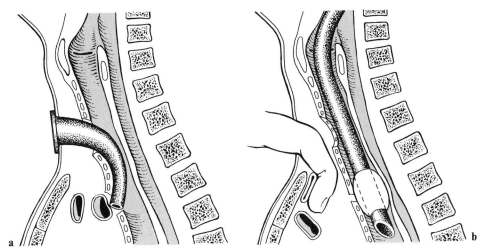

Fig. 1. a An injury caused by a tracheal cannula can give rise to a tracheoarterial fistula. **b** If the bleeding continues after insertion and insufflation of an oral tracheal tube, blind finger dissection is made to compress the brachiocephalic trunk against the sternum

eral arm (Myers et al. 1972; Ramesh and Gazzaniga 1978; Courcy et al. 1985). Jones et al. (1976) used three signs to indicate a satisfactory collateral circulation on innominate artery clamping: (a) the continuation of a right superficial temporal artery pulse or right common carotid artery pulse; (b) absence of change in pupil sizes under light anesthesia; (c) forceful backbleeding from the common carotid artery. If there is doubt about the collateral circulation, however, distal stump pressure can be measured (Bloss and Ward 1980), and if this is low an extra-anatomic reconstruction could be considered, e.g., a bypass from the contralateral common carotid artery. Raskind et al. (1973) recomended permanent occlusion of the innominate artery trunk via a suprasternal approach with placement of a hemostatic clip on the artery. To avoid pneumonitis from aspirated blood, any blood must be carefully removed by irrigation and suction and a fiberoptic bronchoscope should be used to inspect and clean the trachea and the bronchial tree.

Other Vascular Neck Injuries

Seven cases of *arteriovenous fistulas* after thyroidectomy have been reported (Beattie et al. 1960; Downes 1914; French et al. 1959; Ransohoff 1935; Selman 1932; Seror et al. 1967; Webster 1982). The predominating symptom has been a humming sound of high frequency, sometimes to the degree that has caused sleep difficulties. Two of the patients had cardiac incompensation (Selman 1932; Seror et al. 1967). The arteriovenous fistulae were resected with good results and disappearance of the sound sensations. Vollmar (1963) described a patient with a large aneurysm that developed after subtotal thyroidectomy, which he interpreted as the result of a loose ligation causing a "poststenotic" dilatation.

Mora (1929) described an AV fistula between the superior thyroid artery and vein, and Hipona and Harrison (1963) described one between the thyrocervical trunk and internal jugular vein after a prescalene lymph node biopsy. Both produced symptoms in the form of pulsating tumors and were removed leaving no sequelae.

It may be of historical interest to mention the operation with creation of a side-to-side AV fistula between the common carotid artery and internal jugular vein in mentally retarded patients, especially those with juvenile epilepsy, to increase the cerebral circulation with the hope of obtaining better cerebral function. The concept of arterialization of the cerebral venous system was introduced by Sciaroni (1948) and further developed by Beck et al. (1949). Between 1949 and 1953, 363 carotido-jugular fistulas were created in the United States and Europe (Holmes 1964). Adam and Goetz (1970) reported on such patients, who developed cardiac incompensation and in whom the fistula had to be resected. Holmes (1964) had a 12-year follow-up of two patients, one with cardiac insufficiency and the other with hypertension. The symptoms were reversible after repair of the fistulae. Zilkha and Schechter (1969) also reported on a case with cardiac insufficiency 17 years after creation of such a fistula. AV fistulas have been reported in the region of the fascial artery after tonsillectomy (Nova et al. 1972), and after external pin fixation of a mandible fracture (Grelly and Throndson 1944).

After *tonsillectomy* there may be severe hemorrhage, either from lesion of an aberrant carotid artery (Harlowe 1948) or lesion of the external maxillary artery (Gardner 1968). In 1921 there was a dramatic report in the *Journal of the American Medical Association* (anonymous) on the death of a young girl because of fulminant hemorrhage following tonsillectomy, performed by an experienced surgeon who had done more than 500 tonsillectomies without the slightest accident. At the forensic autopsy a large tear was discovered in the internal carotid artery.

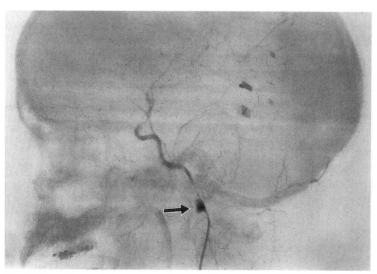

Fig. 2. Carotid pseudoaneurysm after tonsillectomy in a young boy. Ligation of the internal carotid artery was made without sequlae

This lead Schaeffer (1921) to summarize the anatomy of aberrant vessels in surgery of the palatine and pharyngeal tonsils, showing that a tortuous cervical internal carotid artery sometimes protrudes into the pharynx. The carotid artery should be reconstructed whenever possible, whereas ligation of the external maxillary artery is the therapy of choice.

Post-tonsillectomy hemorrhage may also be of a secondary delayed type occurring after more than 24 h, and it may, in rare cases, be catastrophic (Sanderson 1958; Pratt and Root 1960; Utrata 1961). Such hemorrhages are due to defective hemostasis in often relatively small arteries in the tonsillar fossa and are therefore not primarily of vascular surgical concern. Mostly, there is necrotic and infected tissue, making local hemostasis with sutures and stitches difficult and ineffective. In these cases ligation of the external carotid artery as well as of the branches (ascending pharyngeal, superior thyroid, external maxillary, lingual, internal maxillary) may be necessary to prevent backbleeding and to obtain adequate hemostasis. As a late complication after tonsillectomy a pseudoaneurysm may develop (Fig. 2).

In Sweden, among some 15000 tonsillectomies was one fatal bleeding, several weeks after surgery (Ansvarsnämnden 1985). Suture ligation was initially successful, but eventually the carotid artery had to be ligated to stop the recurrent bleedings. Death was due to cerebral infarction from the carotid artery ligation and the shock in connection with a voluminous hemorrhage.

Miller and Bergstrom (1974) reported injuries in two patients after radical neck resection because of malignancies. In the first case there was marked venous congestion and bulbar conjunctivitis 4 years after surgery. At the same time the patient developed first transient ischemic attacks, then a fixed hemiparesis in his right side. Angiography showed a large AV fistula between the carotid artery and the proximal stump of the ligated internal jugular vein. It was considered unresectable and the patient died within a few days. In the other patient left-sided hemiparesis developed 6 days after the radical neck operation. He died, and at autopsy a fresh thrombus was found in the right common artery. Lord (Lord et al. 1958) reported on a patient with laceration of the common carotid carotid artery during a radical neck dissection for laryngeal carcinoma. The carotid artery was ligated, and no sequelae occurred. During a similar operation the subclavian artery was lacerated and transfixed (Lord et al. 1958). Especially in irradiated patients radical neck dissection can cause late problems with infection, pseudoaneurysm formation, and hemorrhage from the large vessels (Sisson et al. 1975).

Delayed hemorrhage because of carotid artery rupture after head and neck tumor surgery is seen almost exclusively in patients who have been irradiated as well (see p. 63). However, there have been reports of three cases were radiation therapy was not given, all with severe infection and occurring 6, 9, and 16 days postoperatively (Ketcham and Hoye 1965; Dibbell et al. 1965). Among 105 consecutive patients undergoing major surgical procedures for head and neck cancer, 46 did not receive radiation therapy and carotid artery necrosis with hemorrhage occurred in none of these, compared with 21% of those who were irradiated in combination with surgery (Joseph and Shumrick 1973).

Friduss et al. (1987) reported a case of innominate artery pseudoaneurysm, after a traffic accident and complicated tracheostomy, which ruptured during dilatation of a chronic subglottic stenosis. The pseudoaneurysm was resected and the distal and proximal part of the innominate artery over sewn; the recovery was complete.

References

Adam YG, Goetz RH (1970) Surgically produced carotid-jugular fistula: 18-year follow-up. Ann Surg 171:93–97

Adolfsson R, Winblad B, Östberg Y (1975) Survival after haemorrhage from the brachiocephalic truncus following tracheostomy. Acta Otolaryngol 80:312–316

Andrews MJ, Pearson FG (1971) Incidence and pathogenesis of tracheal injury following cuffed tube tracheostomy with assisted ventilation: analysis of a two-year prospective study. Ann Surg 773:249–263

Anonymous (1921) The carotid arteries and hemorrhages of the tonsils. JAMA 76:532

Ansvarsnämnden (1985) Unique fatality. Postoperative bleeding after tonsillectomy (in Swedish). Läkartidn 82:2621–2622

Arbulu A, Thoms NW (1974) Tracheal-innominate artery fistula after repair of tracheal stenosis. J Thorac Cardiovasc Surg 67:936–940

Arola MK, Inberg MV, Sotarauta M, Vänttinen E (1979) Tracheoarterial erosion complicating tracheostomy. Ann Chir Gynaecol 68:9–17

Beattie WM, Oldham JB, Ross JA (1960) Superior thyroid arteriovenous aneurysm. Br J Surg 40:456–457

Beck C, McKhann C, Belnap D (1949) Revascularization of the brain through establishment of a cervical arteriovenous fistula. J Pediatr 35:317–329

Bertelsen S, Jensen NM (1987) Innominate artery rupture. A fatal complication of tracheostomy. Ann Chir Gynaecol 76:230–233

Biller HF, Ebert PA (1970) Innominate artery hemorrhage complicating tracheotomy. Ann Otol Rhinol Laryngol 79:301–316

Bloss RS, Ward RE (1980) Survival after tracheoinnominate artery fistula. Am J Surg 139:251–253

Brantigan CO (1973) Delayed major vessel hemorrhage following tracheostomy. J Trauma 13:235–237

Bryant LR, Trinkle JK, Dubilier L (1971) Reappraisal of tracheal injury from cuffed tracheostomy tubes. Experiments in dogs. JAMA 215:625–628

Castaing R, Couraud L, Chomy P, Dumazeau M-M, Favarel-Garrigues J-C (1966) Une complication secondaire rare de la trachéotomie: l'ulcération du tronc artériel brachiocéphalique. J Med Bordeaux 143:1891–1906

Caterine JM (1977) Massive hemorrhage following tracheostomy. J Iowa Med Soc 67:203–206

Ching NPH, Ayres SM, Spina RC, Nealon TF (1974) Endotracheal damage during continuous ventilatory support. Ann Surg 179:123–127

Clin R (1963) Complication d'une scarlatine. Ulcération du tronc brachio-céphalique au 10e jour d'une trachéotomie. Ann Otolaryngol Chir Cervicofac 80:1003–1005

Comer TP, Raskind R, Schmalhorst WR, Arbegast NR (1974) Delayed massive hemorrhage from tracheostomy. J Cardiovasc Surg (Torino) 15:389–391

Conn J, Tolis GA, Shields TW (1969) Fatal hemorrhage following tracheostomy. IMJ 135:27–29

Conrad M, Cameron J, White R (1977) The role of angiography in the diagnosis of tracheal-innominate artery fistula. AJR 128:35–38

Cooper JD (1977) Tracheo-innominate artery fistula: successful management of 3 consecutive patients. Ann Thorac Surg 24:439–447

Couraud L, Castaing R, Laumonier P, Favarel-Garrigue J-C, Bruneteau A (1967) Les hémorragies cataclysmiques tardives des trachéotomisés. Presse Med 75:65–69

Courcy PA, Rodriguez A, Garrett HE (1985) Operative technique for repair of tracheoinnominate artery fistula. J Vasc Surg 2:332–334

Davis JB, Southwick HW (1956) Hemorrhage as a postoperative complication of tracheotomy. Ann Surg 144:893–896

De Montmollin D (1962) Les complications hémorragiques de la trachéotomie. Pract Oto-Rhino-Laryngol 303–309

Deslauriers J, Ginsberg RJ, Nelems JM, Pearson FG (1975) Innominate artery rupture. A major complication of tracheal surgery. Ann Thorac Surg 20:671–677

Dibbell DG, Gowen GF, Shedd DP (1965) Observations on postoperative carotid hemorrhage. Am J Surg 109:765–770

Donovan ST, Ribas A, Blatnik DS, Lehman RH (1977) A late complication of tracheostomy. Wis Med J 76:126–127

Dotzauer G, Althoff H (1966) Pathologische Befunde nach Tracheotomie. Z Prakt Anaesth Wiederbeleb 1:297–305

Downes WA (1914) Arteriovenous aneurysm of the superior thyroid artery and vein. Ann Surg 59:789–790

Duval J-M, Etienne P, Boullier G (1969) Le tronc artériel brachio-céephalique et les hémorragies cataclysmiques de la trachéotomie. Ann Chir 23:437–443

Elstein M, Legg NJ, Murphy M, Park DM, Sutcliffe MML (1971) Guillain-Barré syndrome in pregnancy. Anaesthesia 26:216–224

Engelhardt A (1900) Pathologisch-anatomische und klinische Beiträge zur Frage der Blutungen nach der Tracheotomie wegen Diphtherie im Kindesalter. Mitt Grenzgab Med Chir 6:398–433

Felson B, Cohen S, Courter S, McGuire J (1950) Anomalous right subclavian artery. Radiology 54:340–349

Foltanek C (1892) Über Blutungen nach Tracheotomie bei Diphtheritis. Jahrb Kinderheilkd 33:241–280

Fox JL (1973) Control of common carotid and innominate artery hemorrhage complicating tracheostomy. J Neurosurg 38:394

French WR, Patton RW, Wise RA (1959) Arteriovenous fistula of the superior thyroid artery and vein. Ann Surg 150:149–152

Friduss M, Hoover L, Alessi D, Robertson J (1987) Traumatic innominate pseudoaneurysm rupture during laryngeal dilatation. Ann Oto Rhinol Laryngol 96:695–697

Frühwald F (1885) Casuistische Mitteilungen. Jahrb Kinderheilkd 23:414–417

Gardner J (1968) Sutures and disasters in tonsillectomy. Arch Otolaryngol 88:117–121

Greenway RE (1972) Tracheostomy: surgical problems and complications. Int Anesthesiol Clin 10:151–172

Grelly PW, Throndson AH (1944) Arteriovenous aneurysm resulting from application of Roger Anderson splint. JAMA 124:1128

Grillo H (1975) Discussion to Deslauriers et al. Ann Thorac Surg 20:675–676

Grillo H, Cooper J, Geffin B, Pontoppidan H (1971) A low-pressure cuff for tracheostomy tubes to minimize tracheal injury. A comparative clinical trial. J Thorac Cardiovasc Surg 62:898–907

Gross H, Withalm A (1953) Seltene Arrosionsblutung bei einer tracheotomierten Kehlkopfdiphtherie. Arch Kinderheilkd 147:175–178

Harlowe HD (1948) Complications following tonsillectomy. Laryngoscope 58:861–878

Hewitt RL, Brewer PL, Drapanas T (1970) Aortic arch anomalies. J Thorac Cardiovasc Surg 60:746–753

Hipona FA, Harrison TS (1963) Acquired arteriovenous fistula following prescalene lymph node biopsy. J Thorac Cardiovasc Surg 45:824–826

Holmes T (1964) Circulatory dynamics in the presence of carotid-jugular fistula. Effects of repair after twelve year's patency. Circulation 29:905–910

Hood RM, Rush CE (1962) Lethal hazards of the Mörch respirator. J Thorac Cardiovasc Surg 43:338–342

Ivankovic AD, Thomsen S, Rattenborg CC (1969) Fatal haemorrhage from the innominate artery after tracheostomy. Br J Anaesth 41:450–452

Jarvis JF (1964) Vascular hazards in tracheostomy. J Laryngol Otol 78:781–784

Johnson AC (1951) A fatal hemorrhage due to tracheotomy. J Maine Med Assoc 42:261–262

Jones JW, Reynolds M, Hewitt RL, Drapanas T (1976) Tracheoinnominate artery erosion: successful surgical management of a devastating complication. Ann Surg 184:194–204

Joseph DL, Shumrick DL (1973) Risks for head and neck surgery in previously irradiated patients. Arch Otolaryngol 97:381–384

Kantawala SA, Rege SR, Shah KL (1972) Fatal hemorrhage following tracheostomy. J Postgrad Med 18:156–159

Ketcham AS, Hoye RC (1965) Spontaneous carotid artery hemorrhage after head and neck surgery. Am J Surg 110:649–655

Kia-Noury M, Deubzer W (1963) Tracheotomie in chirurgischer Sicht – ein Erfahrungsbericht. Zentralbl Chir 88:1955–1972

Kmiecik J, Szulc R, Grabus W (1976) Early haemorrhage from brachiocephalic trunk as a complication of tracheostomy. Anaesth Resus Intensive Ther 4:201–204

Körte W (1879) Über einige seltene Nachkrankheiten, nach der Tracheotomie wegen Diphtheritis. Arch Klin Chir 24:238–263

Krejovic B, Jorgacevic D (1971) Clinically undetected aneurysm of inferior thyroid artery and fatal haemorrhage from innominate artery on the eleventh day after tracheotomy (in Russian). Srp Arh Celok Lek 99:177–180

Lane EE, Temes GD, Anderson WH (1975) Tracheal-innominate artery fistula due to tracheostomy. Chest 68:678–683

Langlois J, Logeais Y, Galey J-J, Mathey J (1967) Complications hémorragiques de la trachéotomie: la fissuration du tronc artériel brachio-céphalique dans la trachée. Ann Chir Thor Cardio Vasc 6:443–450

Lewis RJ, Ranade NB (1978) Tracheo-innominate artery fistula. J Med Soc NJ 75:329–331

Lord J, Stone P, Cloutier W, Breidenbach L (1958) Major blood vessel injury during elective surgery. Arch Surg 77:282–288

Lunding M (1964) The tracheotomy tube and postoperative tracheotomy complications. Acta Anaesthesiol Scand 8:181–189

Majeski J, MacMillan B (1978) Tracheo-innominate artery erosion in a burned child. J Trauma 18:137–139

Marcorelli E (1968) Rottura dell'arteria anonima dopo tracheotomia. Nunt Radiologius (Suppl) 1:49–55

Martina A (1963) Die Arrosionsblutungen nach der Tracheotomie durch Canülendecubitus. Dtsch Z Chir 69:567–592

Mathog RH, Kenan PD, Hudson WR (1971) Delayed massive hemorrhage following tracheostomy. Laryngoscope 81:107–119

Mayer J (1957) Tracheotomia inferior, tödliche Arrosionsblutung aus der Arteria anonyma. Monatsschr Ohrenheilkd Laryngol-Rhinol 90:369–372

McDonald JJ, Anson BJ (1940) Variations in the origin of arteries derived from the aortic arch, in American whites and negroes. Am J Phys Anthropol 27:91–103

Mehalic TF, Farhat SM (1972) Tracheoarterial fistula: a complication of tracheostomy in patients with brain stem injury. J Trauma 12:140–143

Miech G, Tempe J-D, Morand G, Otteni J-C, Mantz J-M, Witz J-P (1967) Complications de la trachéotomie – les hémorragies. Ann Chir Thor Cardio Vasc 6:461–463

Miller DR, Bergstrom L (1974) Vascular complications of head and neck surgery. Arch Otolaryngol 100:136–140

Missionznik J (1928) Über tödliche Blutung nach unterer Tracheotomie und Topographie der Arteria anonyma und der Luftröhre. Zentralbl Hals-Nas-Ohrenheilkd 12:175–176

Mora JM (1929) Arteriovenous aneurysm of left superior thyroid vessels. Surg Gynecol Obstet 48:123–124

Mounier-Kuhn P, Rebattu J-P, Haguenauer J-P, Bertrand J, Jacquemard C (1968) Les dangers vasculaires de la trachéotomie. Ann Otolaryngol (Paris) 85:221–228

Mulder DS, Rubush JL (1969) Complications of tracheostomy: relationship to long-term ventilatory assistance. J Trauma 9:389–402

Myers RS, Pilch YH (1969) Temporary control of tracheal-innominate artery fistula. Ann Surg 170:149–151

Myers WO, Lawton BR, Sautter RD (1972) An operation for tracheal-innominate artery fistula. Arch Surg 105:269–274

Neuman O (1974) Untersuchungen zur Entstehung von Tracheal-Schaden als Infektions-Folge bei Langzeit-Intubation. Anaesthesist 23:359–363

Nova S, Tilson D, Stansel H (1972) Arteriovenous fistula secondary to tonsillectomy. Arch Otolaryngol 96:248–249

Nunn DB, Sanchez-Salazar AA, McCullagh JM, Renard A (1975) Trachea-innominate artery fistula following tracheostomy. Ann Thorac Surg 20:698–702

Pathak PN (1969) Rare complication of tracheostomy: erosion of innominate artery. Br Med J 2:426

Pfretzschner C, Kronmesser H-J, Poluda M (1973) Komplikationen nach Tracheotomie. Z Laryngol Rhinol Otol Ihre Grenzgeb 52:616–626

Potondi A (1969) Pathomechanism of haemorrhages following tracheotomy. J Laryngol Otol 83:475–484

Potondi A, Pribilla O (1966) Tödliche Komplikationen bei Tracheotomie. Deutsch Z Gesamte Gerichtl Med 58:40–49

Pratt LW, Root JA (1960) Catastrophic post-tonsillectomy secondary hemorrhage. J Maine Med Assoc 51:7–12

Prenner K, Schroll H, Steiner H (1972) Erfolgreich beherrschte Arrosionsblutung aus dem Truncus brachiocephalicus nach Tracheostomie. Chirurg 43:135–138

Pusterla C (1968) Blutungskomplikationen nach Tracheotomie und deren Verhütung. Schweiz Med Wochenschr 98:979–982

Rabuzzi D, Halsey W, Ikins P, Reed G (1973) Postoperative problems of tracheal resection. Laryngoscope 83:568–575

Ramesh M, Gazzaniga AB (1978) Management of tracheo-innominate artery fistula. J Thorac Cardiovasc Surg 75:138–140

Ransohoff JL (1935) Arteriovenous aneurysm of superior thyroid artery and vein. Surg Gynecol Obstet 61:816–817

Raskind R, Glover MB, Arbegast NR, Comer TP (1973) Control of hemorrhage from the innominate artery complicating tracheostomy through a suprasternal approach. Vasc Surg 7:265–268

Reich MP, Rosenkrantz JG (1968) Fistula between innominate artery and trachea. Arch Surg 96:401–402

Revilla A, Donahoo J, Cameron J (1974) Tracheal-innominate artery fistula after tracheal reconstruction. A case of successful repair. J Thorac Cardiovasc Surg 67:629–633

Rogers L (1969) Complications of tracheostomy. South Med J 62:1496–1500

Rydberg B, Gundersen O, Grumstedt B (1972) Erosion of the innominate artery. Acta Chir Scand 138:537–538

Sanderson BA (1958) Exsanguinating hemorrhage twenty-one days after tonsilloadenoidectomy. Arch Otolaryngol 68:630–631

Schaeffer JP (1921) Aberrant vessels in surgery of the palatine and pharyngeal tonsils. JAMA 77:14–19

Scheldrup EW (1957) Vascular anaomalies of the retro-infrahyoid (pretracheal) space and their importance in tracheotomy. Surg Gynecol Obstet 105:327–331

Schenken JR, Brown JM (1954) Tracheocarotid fistula with fatal hemorrhage following tracheotomy for poliomyelitis. J Pediatr 45:94–97

Schlaepfer K (1924) Fatal hemorrhage following tracheotomy for laryngeal diphtheria. JAMA 82:1581–1583

Sciaroni GH (1948) Reversal of circulation of the brain. Am J Surg 76:150

Selking Ö, Hallén A, Lindholm C-E (1977) Management of the innominate artery haemorrhage – a complication following tracheostomy. Acta Chir Scand 143:489–491

Selman JJ, Freedlander SO (1932) Arteriovenous aneurysm of thyroid vessels. Am J Surg 17:99

Seror J, Mentouri B, Azoulay Cl, Boudjellab O (1967) Anévrysme artérioveineux thyroidien supérieur après thyroidectomie. Mem Acad Chir 93:174–181

Silén W, Spieker D (1965) Fatal hemorrhage from the innominate artery after tracheostomy. Ann Surg 162:1005–1012

Sisson G, Edison B, Bydell D (1975) Transsternal radical neck dissection. Postoperative complications and management. Arch Otolaryngol 101:46–49

Stiles PJ (1965) Tracheal lesions after tracheostomy. Thorax 20:517–522

Subotié R (1963) Arrosionsblutungen nach Eingriffen an der Trachea. Monatsschr Ohrenheilkd Laryngol-Rhinol 97:33–37

Thompson SG (1966) Hazards of tracheostomy. Br Med J 5499:1358

Tilney NL, McArdle CS (1975) Acute lead neuropathy: tracheo-innominate fistula. J R Coll Surg Edinb 20:138–140

Toty L, Hertzog P, Diane C, Aboudi A (1967) Six cas d'hémorrhagie mortelle chez des malades trachéotomisés et placés sous ventilation assistée. Ann Chir Thor Cardio Vasc 6:453–459

Utley JR, Singer MM, Roe BB, Fraser DG, Dedo HH (1972) Definitive management of innominate artery hemorrhage complicating tracheostomy. JAMA 220:577–579

Utrata J (1961) Delayed massive post-tonsillectomy hemorrhage. Eye Ear Nose Throat Mon 40:342–344

Veress L, Romhanyi I (1965) Fatal haemorrhage from the innominate artery after tracheotomy. J Laryngol Otol 79:462–465

Vic-Dupont V, Monsallier J-F, Lissac J, Amstutz P (1967) Les hémorragies par fistulisation du tronc artérial brachio-céphalique chez les trachéotomisés. Ann Chir Thor Cardio Vasc 6:457–470

Vollmar J (1963) Aneurysma der Arteria thyroidea inferior nach Schilddrüsenoperation. Chirurg 34:280–282

von Bihler K, Hutschenreuter K (1966) Tödliche Arrosionsblutungen nach Tracheostomie. Z Prakt Anaesth Wiederbeleb 1:313–319

von der Embe J, Weidenbecher M, Aigner K (1976) Arrosionsblutung nach Tracheotomie. Truncus brachiocephalicus-Ersatz. Chirurg 47:524–526

von Moritz E (1978) Erfolgreich behandelte Arrosionsblutung nach Trachealresektion. Med Klin Wochenschr 90:427–430

von Strauchmann U, Wagemann W (1981) Truncus-brachiocephalicus-Blutung nach Tracheotomie. Zentralbl Chir 106:309–316

Watts J (1963) Tracheostomy in modern practice. Br J Surg 50:954–975

Webster MW (1982) Arteriovenous fistula following thyroidectomy. J Cardiovasc Surg (Torino) 23:515–517

Weiss JB, Ozment KL, Westbrook KC, Williams GD (1976) Tracheal-innominate artery fistula: successful management of two cases. South Med J 69:430–432

Weissman BW (1974) Tracheo-innominate artery fistula. Laryngoscope 84:205–209

Welin F (1964) Hemorrhage from the innominate artery (in Danish). Ugeskr Laeger 126:1079–1081

Willerson JT, Fred HL (1965) Delayed fatal hemorrhage after tracheotomy. Arch Intern Med 116:138–141

Zilkha A, Schechter M (1969) Arteriovenous fistulas of the major vessels of the neck. Acta Radiol [Diagn] (Stockh) 9:560–572

Vascular Complications
of Various General Surgical Procedures

Hernia Repair

Three types of vascular injury may occur following hernia surgery:
1. Bleeding from "corona mortis"
2. Bleeding, pseudoaneurysm, or occlusion from lesion of the common femoral artery
3. Bleeding, stenosis, or thrombosis following lesion or obstruction of the femoral vein

Incidence

The incidence of arterial complications after hernia surgery is not known, but it is probable that they are among the most common and serious arterial injuries occuring in general surgery. The number of published cases is relatively low, however. Natali et al. (1972) published seven cases of their own, and Mèlliere et al. (1980) reviewed 23 cases from the literature, adding two cases of their own. Of 46 cases of iatrogenic vascular injuries reported by Pietri et al. (1981), two were in connection with Bassini hernioplasty.

The incidence of vein injuries is completely unknown. The number of cases published in the literature is very small.

Arterial Lesions

"*Corona mortis*" is a term introduced by Hesselbach, signifying an anatomic variant occurring in about 20% of the population. In these cases the inferior epigastric artery and the obturator artery form a relatively long common branch from the external iliac artery before it divides (Lippert and Pabst 1985). This common branch runs in the lacunar ligament around the origin of the hernia. The anomaly was feared in earlier times, when hernia repair was performed in a more blind fashion than today. Serious bleeding from damage of a "corona mortis" is probably very unusual nowadays.

Lesion of the *common femoral artery* is an important and sometimes serious vascular injury that occurs during hernia repair (Gautier and Bonneton 1972; Mellière et al. 1980; Mendenhall and Fuson 1963; Natali et al. 1972; Niemann et al. 1971; Pillet and Albaret 1973; Shamberger et al. 1984). It is due to deep placement of sutures into the anterior femoral sheath or ileopubic tract. This may cause a tear of the artery, resulting in heavy blood loss or in an arterial stricture following attempts at hemostasis. Macro- or microemboli may originate from the traumatized area, or thrombotic occlusion may develop. At the site of the vascular injury a pseudoaneurysm may form (Smith et al. 1963).

Remarkably enough, the majority of these lesions are not discovered intraoperatively. Occasionally, the only symptom appearing during the operation is a sudden brisk hemorrhage when placing a deep suture to repair the defect in the abdominal wall. Following the operation the patient may develop ischemic symptoms in the affected leg, sometimes with gangrene, but usually only with intermittent claudication. The pseudoaneurysm may be felt as a tender, expanding, pulsating mass in the wound (Elkin 1948), and may rupture after several days or weeks. Infection around the pseudoaneurysm has been reported.

Prophylaxis and Intraoperative Management

The surgeon should identify the artery and the vein and be careful when placing the sutures in this area. The fascial structures should be lifted up when the needle passes to avoid catching the blood vessels in the stitch.

If the surgeon suspects that the needle has gone into the artery he should avoid tying the suture and should immediately withdraw the needle and the thread and apply pressure, enough to arrest the bleeding but not so much that it totally stops the flow in the artery. This maneuver is usually sufficient to achieve hemostasis. Hernia needles are usually quite thick and cutting, however, and damage to the artery may be of such a magnitude that open repair is necessary. In these cases, the artery should be explored to such an extent that arterial clamps can be applied above and below the injury. The arterial sutures can now be placed in a controlled fashion, resulting in arrest of the bleeding without stricture of the artery. Careful postoperative control of the peripheral circulation in the leg is mandatory for early detection of a vascular occlusion.

Late complications such as late occlusion, pseudoaneurysm, or infection are managed according to the general principles of reconstructive vascular surgery. Synthetic grafts may be necessary, as well as extra-anatomic reconstruction from the contralateral femoral artery, or via the foramen obturatum.

Lesions to the Femoral Vein

Constriction of the femoral vein has been described in particular after hernioplasty according to McVay. In this operation, which is considered to have a very low recurrence rate, sutures are placed to adjust the posterior inguinal wall to Cooper's ligament. These sutures should start at the pubic tubercle and continue to the femoral vein. If improperly performed, Cooper's ligament repair can cause constriction of the femoral vein. Nissen (1975) reported on six patients who had painful swelling of the leg following hernia repair according to McVay. In five of them, in whom phlebography was performed, a constriction was found. In two of them a thrombosis was also seen, and pulmonary scintigraphy demonstrated pulmonary emboli. In 1986 Klausner et al. reported three cases of deep venous thrombosis due to obstruction of the femoral vein following McVay repair.

Varicose Vein Surgery

Three types of lesions have been reported following surgery for varicose veins:
1. Ligation or resection of the femoral vein (Baumann 1978; Luke and Miller 1948; Tera 1967)
2. Ligation, resection, or stripping of the common, superficial, and deep femoral arteries (Cockett 1986; Eger et al. 1973; Luke and Miller 1948; Pegoraro et al. 1987)
3. Injection of sclerosing agents into arteries, either during surgery, or during percutaneous sclerotherapy (Cockett 1986; Tournay 1970)

Incidence

The incidence of serious vascular complications to varicose vein surgery is not known. Natali (1979) reported 12 cases in a series of 125 vascular injuries occurring after various types of surgery. Altogether 15 cases of injury, mostly to the femoral vein, have been reported to the Swedish Board of Health and Welfare during the past 20 years. The incidence of such lesions may therefore be relatively high, even considering the large number of such operations performed.

Arterial Lesions

Most of the vascular lesions following varicose vein surgery that are documented in the literature concern the arteries. Surprisingly enough, the femoral arteries can be mistaken for the saphenous vein, even by a surgeon who is careful and experienced. Severe spasm may obviously completely eliminate pulsations. The lesions may be either ligation or resection of the common femoral artery, superficial femoral artery, or deep femoral artery, or even stripping of the femoral artery down to the popliteal artery or to the tibial artery (Eger et al. 1973; Leitz and Schmidt 1974; Liddicoat et al. 1975; Pegoraro et al. 1987). Occasionally, sclerosing agents have also been injected into the arterial system intraoperatively (see p. 159).

Remarkably, the diagnosis of an arterial lesion is usually delayed for several hours or even weeks. The impaired circulation in the affected extremity is often ascribed to "spasm." Cockett (1986) reported nine cases of arterial injury during varicose vein surgery, three with stripping of the artery, the others with ligation or resection. In none of them was the error recognized at the time of the original operation. Consequently, only one patient had restoration to his preoperative status while all the others had serious sequelae, either with claudication, pain at rest, or amputation (three patients). Natali (1979) reported on five arterial lesions, all of them requiring amputation, again essentially due to delayed diagnosis.

Prophylaxis and Management

Arterial lesions seem to occur even when the operation is performed by an experienced surgeon. It is difficult to give general advice on how to avoid arterial injuries. It is important, however, for every surgeon to be aware of the possibility of such an injury, in order to recognize it as soon as possible. Any sign of peripheral ischemia, such as paleness, pain, paresthesia, or paresis therefore requires immediate and careful clinical examination, including palpation of peripheral pulses. Early exploration, if necessary after angiography or with intraoperative angiography, is mandatory.

Reconstructive arterial surgery is usually not particularly difficult. Even patients who have undergone stripping of the femoral, popliteal, and tibial arteries down to the ankle have been successfully handled with reconstructive surgery, using combined saphenous vein and synthetic grafts.

Venous Lesions

According to the reports to the Swedish Board of Health and Welfare, lesions of the femoral vein are more common than arterial lesions during varicose vein surgery. Only a few such cases are reported in the literature, however.

In contrast to arterial lesions, most venous lesions are caused by unexperienced surgeons, and they are discovered intraoperatively. Usually, there is a sudden venous hemorrhage during the dissection in the groin, sometimes massive enough to cause the death of the patient. Very often the surgeon places arterial forceps deep into the operative field in an effort to achieve hemostasis and thereby damages vital structures, particularly the femoral vein. It is therefore often necessary to resect and reconstruct the damaged vein.

Prophylaxis and Management

In our experience, most venous injuries are caused by young surgeons who have not had good training or are not well assisted. An important step in decreasing the risk of venous injuries is therefore to provide good training to young surgeons, and to give them good assistence during their first experience of this type of surgery. They should also be instructed to avoid using arterial forceps blindly, thereby causing more damage to vital structures. If there is a massive venous hem-

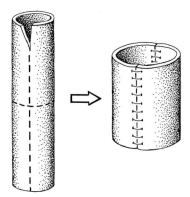

Fig. 1. A useful technique to reconstruct the femoral vein. The saphenous vein is usually too narrow to be directly used as a substitute. Two segments of the saphenous vein are therefore split longitudinally and sewn together along the longitudinal margins, giving rise to a graft of twice the circumference

orrhage, it should be arrested temporarily by elevation and compression, and a senior surgeon should be called in.

When a damaged part of the femoral vein has to be resected it is often necessary to replace it with a vein transplant. The saphenous vein, if necessary from the contralateral leg, is useful, but only if it is cut longitudinally and sutured, thereby doubling the circumference of the vein (Fig. 1). This procedure usually creates a transplant with the same diameter as the femoral vein (Tera 1967). Even so, there is an obvious risk of occlusion of the femoral vein, particularly during the first few weeks after the reconstruction. A distal arteriovenous shunt can be used temporarily to decrease this risk. As an alternative, the patient can be heparinized, and heparinization should be followed by treatment with oral anticoagulants for several weeks. If there are signs of rethrombosis a re-exploration should be performed.

Intraarterial Injection
of Sclerosing Agents During Varicose Vein Treatment

In some patients in whom the femoral artery has been mistaken for the saphenous vein, sclerosing agents have been injected into the artery. This has almost invariably resulted in gangrene and amputation.

Several cases have been described where there has been an accidental intra-arterial injection during percutaneous sclerotherapy for varicose veins. In 1970 Tournay described a patient in whom an injection into an artery in the calf caused ischemia and muscle necrosis, and Buri reported a case in which a sclerosing agent was injected into a patient's posterior tibial artery behind the medial malleolus, resulting in sloughing of soft tissues and osteomyelitis of the calcaneus. In 1971 Martin and Eastcott described a case of intra-arterial injection behind the medial malleolus. Despite treatment with heparin and low-molecular-weight dextran there was ischemic damage to the first and second toes with tissue necrosis. In 1974 Fegan and Pegum presented five cases of accidental intra-arterial injection of sodium tetradecylsulfate during treatment of varicose veins. Severe ischemia and gangrene occurred in two of the cases. Fegan and Pegum recommended heparin and low-molecular-weight dextran in the management of these patients. They pointed out that symptoms resulting from the intra-arterial injection may not occur immediately, but may be delayed for several hours.

Abdominal Surgery

Several types of vascular injury occur after abdominal surgery. The following three are the most important:
1. Lesion of hepatic arteries
2. Arterioportal fistula
3. Damage to the blood supply to abdominal organs

Lesions of Hepatic Arteries

Lesion of the hepatic artery has been a well-known complication to abdominal surgery since the beginning of this century. Due to difficulties in reconstructing the lesions, they usually result in ligation or, more rarely, in the formation of aneurysm or pseudoaneurysm. The consequences of hepatic artery ligation have long been debated. It is known that only about one third of the total hepatic blood flow comes via the hepatic artery, the rest coming from the portal system. Furthermore, the oxygen content of the portal blood is slightly higher than that of the blood in the systemic circulation. Harberer (1905) was one of the first to study the consequences of hepatic artery ligation. In experiments with dogs he observed that ligation distal to the gastroduodenal artery resulted in severe hepatic necrosis, while ligation proximal to that branch usually had no harmful sequelae, due to the better collateral circulation. In a classic report by Graham and Cannell (1933), 27 cases of hepatic artery ligation were collected from the literature. In this clinical study as well the site of ligation was found to be important. Ligation of the common hepatic artery seemed to take place without impairment of hepatic nutrition. Ligation of the proper hepatic artery before the origin of the right gastric artery could also be undertaken without ill effects (Popper 1953). Ligation beyond this point was usually found to be accompanied by widespread hepatic necrosis, but it can be made with survival (Edgecombe and Gardner 1951). Ligation of the right or left hepatic artery was also found to cause hepatic necrosis in the affected area. The considerable anatomic variation in arterial supply of the liver must be remembered (Postlethwait et al. 1964).

The Graham and Cannell study, which had a great impact on surgeons for many years, also demonstrated a frightfully high overall mortality after hepatic artery ligation, amounting to almost 60%. In their report, only three patients had the common hepatic artery ligated, seven the proper hepatic artery, seven the right hepatic artery, and eight the left hepatic artery. In two cases the site of ligation was unknown. It is obvious, however, from an analysis of Graham's and Cannell's cases, that severe blood loss and more or less pronounced hemorrhagic shock was present in most of the patients. This obviously contributed to the mortality (Brittain et al. 1964).

The cause of death following hepatic artery ligation has been discussed extensively. Markowitz et al. (1949) found that the mortality in dogs could be decreased considerably by administering penicillin, supporting their hypothesis that bacterial invasion was an important cause of death. It has been pointed out, however, that, in contrast to the dog liver, the human liver is sterile, and the importance of penicillin administration in human beings is still unclear.

During the past several decades our attitude to hepatic artery lesions has changed. Several reports on hepatic artery ligation during surgery for complicated bile duct problems, or for gastroduodenal ulcer or tumor, have demonstrated that the mortality is low. Although it is obvious that there is some ischemia of the liver, widespread liver necrosis is rare. It has been demonstrated that extraction of oxygen from the portal venous blood increases with occlusion of the hepatic artery, thereby compensating for some of the loss of arterial supply. The signs of liver ischemia are usually limited to slight and temporary increases of S-GOT, S-GPT, and LDH.

The use of hepatic artery ligation as one of the steps in the treatment of hepatic tumors has confirmed the safety of the procedure. A number of cases of hepatic artery occlusion have also occurred following long-term catheterization of the hepatic artery for chemotherapy, resulting in hepatic artery thrombosis (Lucas et al. 1971). A less common consequence of a hepatic artery lesion is formation of a pseudoaneurysm which communicates with the bile ducts, causing hematobilia.

Hepatic artery pseudoaneurysm may occur after various surgical procedures such as cholecystectomy (Guida and Moore 1966; Harlaftis and Akin 1977; Thomas and May 1981).

Arterioportal Fistula

It is well known that arteriovenous fistula may occur after any kind of surgery outside the abdominal cavity. Similarly, surgery inside the abdominal cavity may result in arterioportal fistula.

Incidence and Occurrence

Around 30% of all arterioportal fistulae are considered to be iatrogenic, the remaining being post-traumatic or congenital (Beduhn and Vollmar 1970). They may occur after any type of surgery in the abdomen (Linder et al. 1968) such as of the gallbladder and bile ducts (Pridgen and Jacobs 1962), stomach (Blanckwell and Whelan 1965; Bugge-Asperheim et al. 1980; Clot et al. 1980; Dalichau and Schneider 1968; Geremia et al. 1985; Korobkin et al. 1973; Langsam and Hermann 1965; Morand et al. 1973; Nolan et al. 1974; Reams 1960; Thurston et al. 1977; Rueff et al. 1969; Yeo and Ernst 1986; van der Heyde and Vink 1966), small intestine (Durham et al. 1962; Grafe and Steinberg 1966; Movitz and Finne 1966; Munnell et al. 1960; Tibell et al. 1987), large intestine (Currin and Metcalf 1966) and spleen (Buchholz 1949).

The true incidence of this complication is not known. The condition was first described in 1886 by Weigert. In 1971 van Way et al. reported 57 cases collected from the English-language literature.

Symptoms and Management

The *symptoms* of an arterioportal fistula are different from those of other types of arteriovenous fistulae. Most important is the portal hypertension produced by the fistula, resulting in hematemesis or ascites in 16 of the 57 cases reviewed by van Way et al. (1971). In contrast to arteriovenous fistulae, congestive heart failure and circulatory overload seem to be relatively uncommon, observed in only ten of their cases. Other authors have claimed that circulatory overload never occurs in an arterioportal fistula due to the so-called hepatic protection, which was studied experimentally by Mooney and co-workers (1970). They demonstrated that when the liver is interposed between an experimental arteriovenous fistula and the heart, the elevated cardiac output drops to almost control value. Clinical experience seems to support the experimental study and indicates that circulatory overload, although it occasionally occurs with an arterioportal fistula, is much less common than with arteriovenous fistulae.

In all reports, abdominal pain is a predominating symptom of arterioportal fistula. The reason for this is not quite clear, but it is obvious that in most cases it is cured by operation. Diarrhea is also a relatively common complaint of these patients which is not readily explained. The key to the diagnosis is often the finding of a machinery murmur over the abdomen. Occasionally, this murmur is the only symptom in an otherwise asymptomatic patient. The diagnosis can be confirmed with angiography. Recently the use of computerized tomography has been described (Beck and Daniel 1988).

Surgical *treatment* consists of resecting the fistula. The results of this treatment have in the majority of cases been completely satisfactory. Interestingly enough, however, in some of the patients portal hypertension remains, and sometimes hematemesis and/or ascites recur. It has been suggested that a long-standing arterioportal fistula may cause portal fibrosis which may remain after the correction of the fistula.

Damage to the Blood Supply to Abdominal Organs

Arteries

The three major arteries – the celiac artery and the superior and inferior mesenteric arteries – may be damaged during selective catheterization (see p. 8) but rarely during surgical procedures. An exception is the inferior mesenteric artery, which often has to be sacrificed during aortic surgery. The important problem of intestinal ischemia following ligation of the inferior mesenteric artery is discussed in textbooks on vascular surgery and will not be presented here.

Lesions of the superior mesenteric artery have been described after extensive tumor surgery, particularly for retroperitoneal tumors. In 1970 Ikard and Merendino described a patient with a retroperitoneal neurofibroma. During its removal, an artery was divided which about 2 h later was found to be the superior mesenteric artery. The circulation to the small intestine was re-established with a dacron graft from the aorta to the distal end of the divided artery. In 1985 Sirinek and Levine described 25 patients with traumatic injuries of the proximal superior mesenteric vessels. Only one case was iatrogenic, consisting in a patient who sustained an injury during a diagnostic laparoscopy. In 1981 Boontje described a case of injury to the superior mesenteric artery during pancreaticoduodenectomy for cancer.

A special problem in abdominal surgery is injury to the collateral circulation of the intestine. It is well known that following chronic occlusion of one, two, or even all three of the arteries to the intestinal tract the circulation can be sustained as a result of an extensive collateral circulation. These collaterals form large, tortuous vessels, so-called meandering vessels, to the intestinal tract (Moskowitz et al. 1964). These vessels (the artery of Drummond, the arch of Riolan, and the arch of Treves; Moskowitz et al. 1964) may be accidently divided during abdominal surgery, or they may have to be sacrificed. However, the flow capacity in these vessels does not seem to be very large. Buchardt Hansen (1977) measured the flow in four patients with occluded superior mesenteric arteries and a Riolan's arcade from the inferior to the superior mesenteric artery. The flow was 36, 40, 56, and

192 ml/min respectively, which is very low compared with the total blood flow of the intestinal tract, which exceeds 1000 ml. Little is known about the risk of dividing these vessels.

Veins

Superior mesenteric vein thrombosis is rarely iatrogenic. In 1968 Mergenthaler and Harris described one patient in whom a pancreatoduodenectomy was complicated by a superior mesenteric vein thrombosis. At the end of the operation the small bowel was edematous and cyanotic. A fresh thrombus was found in the superior mesenteric vein and was removed, resulting in restoration of the circulation.

Vascular Lesions in Other Types of General Surgery

Practically every type of general surgery can result in vascular injury, particularly in an arteriovenous fistula after mass or suture ligation (Fig. 2). Here are a few examples:

Sternotomy, which is used with increasing frequency in open heart surgery, may result in an arteriovenous fistula between the internal mammary artery and vein or a pseudoaneurysm (Deuvaert et al. 1987; Longmaid et al. 1980; Maher et al. 1982; Martin et al. 1973). This lesion may be caused by the sternal wire used to close the incision.

Pericardiocentesis with an indwelling pericardial catheter has also been reported to result in an internal mammary arteriovenous fistula.

Thoracocentesis may result in damage of the phrenic vessels with formation of an arteriovenous fistula (Elkin 1949; Silverstein et al. 1978).

Radical mastectomy may result in an arteriovenous fistula between the internal mammary artery and vein (Glenn and Steinberg 1959). Damage to the axillary

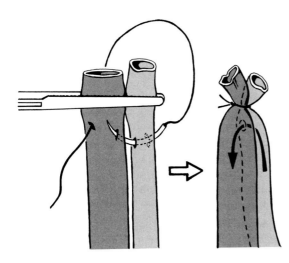

Fig. 2. Suture ligation of an artery and a vein causing the development of an arteriovenous fistula

arteries and veins has also been reported following this operation (Lord et al. 1958). The arterial lesion has been treated with direct anastomosis or grafting (Lord et al. 1958).

References

Baumann G (1978) Arterien- und Venenverletzungen bei Saphenektomien – deren Verhütung und Therapie. Ergeb Angiologi 18:245–250

Beck B, Daniel H (1988) Iatrogene mesenteriale AV-Fistel nach Magenresektion. Fortschr Röntgenstr 148:89–90

Beduhn D, Vollmar J (1970) Arterio-portale Fistel nach Magenresektion. Radiologe 10:304–309

Blackwell TL, Whelan TJ (1965) Arteriovenous fistula as a complication of gastrectomy. Am J Surg 109:197–200

Boontje H (1981) Iatrogenic vascular trauma. Vasc Surg 15:266–271

Brittain RS, Marchioro TL, Hermann G, Wadell WR, Starzl TE (1964) Accidental hepatic artery ligation in humans. Am J Surg 107:822–832

Buchardt Hansen HJ (1977) Chronic and acute intestinal ischemia (in Danish). Fadl's forlag, Kopenhagen

Buchholtz RR (1949) Arteriovenous fistula of the splenic vessels. Report of a case following splenectomy. Ann Surg 149:590–592

Bugge-Asperheim B, Svennevig JL, Birkeland S (1980) Arterio-venous fistula following partial gastrectomy. Ann Chir Gynaecol 69:119–121

Buri P (1970) Versehentliche Injektion der Arteria tibialis posterior bei der Krampfaderverödung. Praxis 59:924–927

Clot J-P, Bouchon J-P, Calmat A, Bussone M (1980) Les fistules artério-veineuses postgastrectomie. A propos d'une nouvelle observation. J Chir (Paris) 117:247–251

Cockett FB (1986) Arterial complications during surgery and sclerotherapy of varicose veins. Phlebologie 1:3–6

Curring JF, Metcalf BH (1966) Postcolectomy arteriovenous fistula. Report of a case. Am J Gastroenterol 46:352–355

Dalichau H, Schneider V (1968) Iatrogene arterioportale Fisteln. Chir Prax 12:219–226

Deuvaert FE, Dumont N, van Nooten G, De Paepe J, Primo G (1987) Poststernotomy arteriovenous fistula of internal mammary origin with pseudoaneurysmal subcutaneous extension. J Cardiovasc Surg (Torino) 28:343–344

Durham M, Robnett A, Harper H, Yekel R (1962) Arteriovenous fistula of the mesenteric vessels. West J Surg Obstet Gynecol 70:9–11

Edgecombe PW, Gardner C (1951) Accidental ligation of the hepatic artery and its treatment. Can Med Assoc J 64:518–522

Eger M, Golcman L, Torok G, Hirsch M (1973) Inadvertent arterial stripping in the lower limb: problems of management. Surgery 73:23–27

Elkin DC (1948) Aneurysm following surgical procedures. Report of five cases. Ann Surg 127:769–779

Elkin DC (1949) Arteriovenous aneurysm of the phrenic vessels. JAMA 141:531–532

Fegan WG, Pegum JM (1974) Accidental intra-arterial injection during sclerotherapy of varicose veins. Br J Surg 61:124–126

Gautier R, Bonneton G (1972) Deux observations de lésions artérielles au cours de la cure de hernie inguinale. Chirurgie 98:722–723

Geremia U, Nicodemo P, Grazia M, Caprioli F (1985) Contributo allo studio delle fistole artero-venose iatrogene celiaco-mesenteriche; in relazione ad una nuova osservazione di fistola artero-venosa post-gastrectomia. Chir Ital 37:57–71

Glenn F, Steinberg I (1959) Arteriovenous fistula of the right internal mammary vessels following radical mastectomy: visualization by angiocardiography. J Thorac Surg 33:719–722

Grafe WR, Steinberg I (1966) Superior mesenteric arteriovenous fistula following small-bowel resection. Gastroenterology 51:231–235

Graham RR, Cannell D (1933) Accidental ligation of the hepatic artery. Report of one case, with a review of the cases in the literature. Br J Surg 20:566–578

Guida PM, Moore SW (1966) Aneurysm of the hepatic artery. Report of five cases with a brief review of the previously reported cases. Surgery 60:299–310

Harberer H (1905) Experimentelle Unterbindung der Leberarterie. Langenbecks Arch Klin Chir 78:557–587

Harlaftis NN, Akin JT (1977) Hemobilia from ruptured hepatic artery aneurysm. Am J Surg 133:229–232

Ikard R, Merendino KA (1970) Accidental excision of the superior mesenteric artery. Surg Clin North Am 50:1075–1085

Klausner JM, Noveck H, Skornick Y, Lelcuk S, Rozin RR (1986) Femoral vein occlusion following McVay repair. Postgrad Med J 62:301–302

Korobkin M, Kantor I, Pollard J et al. (1973) Arteriovenous fistula between systemic and portal circulations following partial gastrectomy. Diagn Radiol 109:311–314

Langsam LB, Hermann RE (1965) Postgastrectomy arteriovenous fistula of the gastroduodenal vessels. Report of a case. Cleve Clin Q 32:29–33

Leitz KH, Schmidt FC (1974) Iatrogene Arterienverletzung bei Babcockscher Venenexhairese. Vasa 3:45–49

Liddicoat JE, Bekassy SM, Daniell MB, De Bakey ME (1975) Inadvertent femoral artery "stripping": surgical management. Surgery 77:318–320

Linder F, Vollmar J, Krumhaar D (1968) Die arterio-venösen Fisteln des Pfortadergebietes. Langenbecks Arch Klin Chir 320:50–63

Lippert H, Pabst R (1985) Arterial variations in man. Classification and frequency. Bergmann, Munich

Longmaid HE, Jay M, Phillips D (1980) Angiographic evaluation of post-sternotomy arteriovenous fistula of the internal mammary artery and vein. Cardiovasc Intervent Radiol 3:150–152

Lord JM, Stone PW, Cloutier WA, Breidenbach L (1958) Major blood vessel injury during elective surgery. Arch Surg 77:282–288

Lucas RJ, Tumacder O, Wilson GS (1971) Hepatic artery occlusion following hepatic artery catheterization. Ann Surg 173:238–243

Luke JC, Miller GG (1948) Disasters following the operation of ligation and retrograde injection of varicose veins. Ann Surg 127:426–431

Maher TD, Glenn JF, Magovern GJ (1982) Internal mammary arteriovenous fistula after sternotomy. Arch Surg 117:1100–1101

Markowitz J, Rappaport AM, Scott AC (1949) Prevention of liver necrosis following ligation of hepatic artery. Proc Soc Exp Biol Med 70:305

Martin A, Ross BA, Braimbridge MV (1973) Peristernal wiring in closure of median sternotomy. J Thorac Cardiovasc Surg 66:145–146

Martin PGC, Eastcott HHG (1971) Sclerosant injection for varicose veins. Br Med J 4:555

Mellière D, Dermer J, Danis RK, Becquemin JP, Renaud J (1980) Complications artérielles de la chirurgie inguinale. Intéret du remplacement veineux in situ. J Chir (Paris) 117:531–535

Mendenhall E, Fuson R (1963) Femoral artery injury during inguinal herniorrhaphy. JAMA 186:731–732

Mergenthaler FW, Harris MN (1968) Superior mesenteric vein thrombosis complicating pancreatoduodenectomy: successful treatment by thrombectomy. Ann Surg 167:106–111

Mooney CS, Honaker AD, Griffen WO (1970) Influence of the liver on arteriovenous fistulas. Arch Surg 100:154–156

Morand P, Potier N, Barsotti J, Raynaud R (1973) Hypertension portale par aneurysme arterio-veineux des vaisseaux gastro-epiploiques droits après gastrectomie. Sem Hôp Paris 49:1837–1843

Moskowitz M, Zimmerman H, Felson B (1964) The meandering mesenteric artery of the colon. AJR 92:1088–1099

Movitz D, Finne B (1960) Preoperative arteriovenous aneurysm in mesentery after small-bowel resection. JAMA 173:126–128

Munnell ER, Mota CR, Thompson WB (1960) Iatrogenic arteriovenous fistula: report of a case involving the superior mesenteric vessels. Am Surg 26:738–744

Natali J, Benhamou AC (1979) Iatrogenic vascular injuries. A review of 125 cases (excluding angiographic injuries). J Cardiovasc Surg (Torino) 20:169–176

Natali J, Kieffer E, Maraval M, Lacombe M, Poullain J-C (1972) Accidents artériels au cours du traitement chirurgical des hernies de l'aine. Chirurgie 98:517–524

Niemann F, Kovacicek S, Sailer R (1971) Gefäßverletzungen bei Leisten- und Schenkelbruchoperationen. Chirurgische Sorgfaltspflicht und Kriterien schuldhaften Verhaltens. Zentralbl Chir 96:408–412

Nissen HM (1975) Constriction of the femoral vein following inguinal hernia repair. Acta Chir Scand 141:279–281

Nolan T, Grady E, Crumbley AJ (1974) Systemic-portal arteriovenous fistula: a case report. J Med Ass Georgia 63:310–311

Pegoraro M, Baracco C, Ferrero F, Palladino F (1987) Successful vascular reconstruction after inadvertent femoral artery "stripping". J Cardiovasc Surg (Torino) 28:440–444

Pietri P, Alagni G, Settembrini PG, Gabrielli F (1981) Iatrogenic vascular lesions. Int Surg 66:213–216

Pillet J, Albaret P (1973) A propos des accidents artériels au cours du traitment chirurgical des hernies de l'aine. Chirurgie 99:210–213

Popper HL (1953) Ligation of accidentally torn hepatic artery. Am J Surg 85:113–115

Postlethwait RW, Hernandez RR, Dillon ML (1964) Hepatic artery lesions. Ann Surg 159:895–910

Preger L (1967) Hepatic arteriovenous fistula after percutaneous liver biopsy. AJR 101:619

Pridgen WR, Jacobs JK (1962) Postoperative arteriovenous fistula. Surgery 51:205–206

Reams GB (1960) A middle colic arteriovenous fistula developing as a postgastrectomy complication. Arch Surg 81:757–760

Rueff FL, Bedacht R, Becker HM, Heinze HG (1969) Arterio-venöse Fistel nach Magenresektion. Münch Med Wochenschr 111:185–187

Shamberger RC, Ottinger LW, Malt RA (1984) Arterial injuries during inguinal herniorrhaphy. Ann Surg 200:83–85

Silverstein R, Crumbo D, Long DL, Kokko JP, Hull AR, Vergne-Marini P (1978) Iatrogenic arteriovenous fistula. An unusual complication of indwelling pericardial catheter and intrapericardial steroid instillation for the treatment of uremic pericarditis. Arch Intern Med 138:308–310

Smith RF, Szilagyi DE, Pfeifer JR (1963) Arterial trauma. Arch Surg 86:825–835

Tera H (1967) Emergency repair of femoral vein accidentally divided at operation for varicose veins. Acta Chir Scand 133:283–287

Thomas WEG, May RE (1981) Hepatic artery aneurysm following cholecystectomy. Postgrad Med J 57:393–395

Thurston JB, Milan MF, Winegarner FC (1977) Iatrogenic fistula of the gastroduodenal vessels. J Indiana State Med Assoc 70:233–235

Tibell A, Hallböök T, Ryden L, Puskar W (1987) Arteriovenous fistula – uncommon complication after small bowel resection (in Swedish) Läkartidningen 84:2505–2506

Tournay R (1970) Les injections intra-artérielles fortuites de substances schlérogènes. Phlebologie 22:117–118

van der Heyde MN, Vink M (1966) A patient with an iatrogenous arteriovenous fistula in the territory of the portal vein. Arch Chir Neerl 18:267–271

van Way CW, Crane JM, Riddell DH, Foster JH (1971) Arteriovenous fistula in the portal circulation. Surgery 70:876–890

Wallace S, Medellin H, Nelson RS (1972) Angiographic changes due to needle biopsy of the liver. Diagn Radiol 105:13–18

Weigert C (1886) In die Milzvene geborstenes Aneurysma einer Milzarterie. Virchows Arch Path Anat 104:26

Yeo CJ, Ernst CB (1986) Arteriovenous fistulas after gastrectomy: case report and review of the literature. Surgery 99:505–510

Pediatric Vascular Injuries

Types of Injury

Umbilical arterial catheterization may cause vessel wall perforation or avulsion with bleeding; vascular occlusion, in the form of (a) thrombosis with aortoiliac or visceral artery occlusion, (b) thrombosis with microembolization, or (c) Wharton's jelly embolization; injury by a foreign body from a broken catheter; or late sequelae such as mycotic aneurysm, a renal artery occlusion with renovascular hypertension, or intermittent claudication and impaired growth. Injuries caused by arteriography, heart catheterization, or arterial puncture will be discussed in this chapter only when they involve special problems concerning children. Otherwise the reader is referred to p. 8. Injuries also occur during surgical procedures.

Review articles concerning vascular injuries in children have been written by Smith and Green (1981) and by Flanigan and Schuler (1987). Special reviews on umbilical artery catheterization have been published by Wesström (1979) and Thompson et al. (1980).

Special Problems Concerning Iatrogenic Vascular Trauma in Children

The size of the vessels in children is much smaller than in adults. In neonates a 2-F Fogarty catheter passes through the common femoral artery (Flanigan et al. 1983). Small arteries are fragile, with thin walls and weak support from surrounding structures. When femoral arteries are catheterized complications are relatively common in youngsters but are seldom seen after about the age of 8–10 years (Freed et al. 1974; Jacobsson et al. 1980; Mortensson et al. 1975 a; Mortensson 1976; Hohn et al. 1969). Children have been found to have a more rapid collateral development than adults (Mortensson 1976).

Arteries in children, especially the very young, have a great tendency to develop spasm, (Boijsen and Lundström 1968; Mortensson et al. 1975 a; Mortensson 1976; Richardson et al. 1981; O'Neill 1983). In the study by Mortensson et al. (1975 b) plethysmographic arterial peak flow was diminished in children below 9 years of age on the catheterized side after arterial as well as venous catheterization but returned to normal on the following day. If pulses have not returned 3–8 h after femoral artery catheterization, however, there is almost always a thrombotic occlusion (White et al. 1968; Mansfield et al. 1970). With a decrease in flow the tendency to spasm may increase the risk of thrombosis development. The tendency to spasm also makes arterial surgery in children technically more difficult (Smith and Green 1981).

Those children who most require umbilical artery catheters are also the ones most predisposed to thromboembolic complications. They often have a low cardiac output, polycythemia, hyperosmolarity, and a high hematocrit. Newborn infants have a relative polycythemia and hyperviscosity which can be aggravated because of a tendency to rapid dehydration during various diseases. Infants of diabetic mothers may have severe hyperviscosity (O'Neill 1983). Catheterization is often performed in children with cardiac diseases, who have a relative polycythemia for that reason. Children with a high hematocrit have a marked reduction in plethysmographically measured arterial peak flow after femoral artery catheterization and also more thrombotic occlusions (Mortensson et al. 1975a).

Henriksson et al. (1979) reported that severely ill newborns had low antithrombin-III levels and high factor-VIII activity. Tyson et al. (1976) found that standard coagulation studies provided little help in predicting, diagnosing, or monitoring the development of arterial thrombosis. In five cases of umbilical artery catheter-induced thrombosis, however, there was no decrease in fibrinolytic activity in the aorta. The small vascular volume in children leaves small margin for volume alterations, and a low-flow state can therefore rapidly develop, a situation which increases the thrombogenicity.

Goldblom et al. (1967) called attention to a particular situation when the attempt to perform femoral venipuncture becomes hazardous. Three small children who were edematous because of an idiopathic nephrotic syndrome developed arterial thrombosis with gangrene, leading to amputation. The same phenomenon has been described in severely dehydrated children (Polesky and Harvey 1968).

The inability to communicate verbally makes the diagnosis of ischemia especially difficult in small children. In cases of ischemia, diagnostic arteriography should be avoided because of the high rate of complications which might aggravate the ischemic state. If an umbilical artery catheter has been inserted, however, angiography can be performed before pull-out of the catheter. Other diagnostic modalities are B-mode scan, nuclear aortography, and computerized subtraction angiography. The rapidly developing ultrasonographic techniques in particular will be of great diagnostic importance.

Long-term sequelae may also develop in patients who are asymptomatic when the acute thrombotic occlusion occurs, in the form of impaired growth of the extremities. Therefore, a careful long-term follow-up is important.

Incidence

In many series on vascular trauma in children iatrogenic injuries are the most common, at least in the younger age groups. Table 1 shows recalculated data from two publications, with a clear relationship between age and proportion of iatrogenic trauma.

There are, however, variations in the number of iatrogenic injuries in various publications. Thus, in a series from Houston, 1957–1977, there were three iatrogenic and 50 noniatrogenic injuries (Meagher et al. 1979), and from Louisville five were iatrogenic and 24 noniatrogenic (Richardson et al. 1981). Shaker et al. (1976) from Johns Hopkins and Whitehouse et al. (1976) from Ann Arbor had

Table 1. Percent of iatrogenic arterial injuries in relation to patient age

Age (years)	Number of injuries		Percent iatrogenic	
	O'Neill (1983)	Shaker et al. (1976)	O'Neill (1983)	Shaker et al. (1976)
<2	27	14	81	86
2–6	30	21	43	57
>6	53	36	36	47

incidences of 58% and 57% respectively. Leblanc et al. (1985) from Toronto reported 40 iatrogenic injuries from a total of 48 (83%): 35 after heart catheterization, two after femoral artery cannulation during extracorporeal circulation, two from femoral artery monitoring, and one after subclavian flap repair in a case of aortic coarctation. Klein et al. (1982) reported 33 injuries in 32 patients: 21 after angiography, seven after umbilical artery catheterization, two after radial artery cannulation, and one each after spinal fusion, cardiopulmonary bypass, and birth trauma. The classification of the last one as iatrogenic may be a matter for discussion. In this series 21 injuries were considered to have been caused by mechanical trauma and were operated on. Eighteen occlusions were caused by thrombosis, two were due to compressing hematomas, and one was due to aortic distortion after posterior spinal fusion. The others were treated conservatively, the symptoms disappeared, and they were considered to have been due to spasm. In six cases (18%) there was tissue loss as an end result. Flanigan et al. (1983) collected a large number of iatrogenic injuries (79 in 76 children) – as in other publications, mostly induced by transfemoral cardiac catheterization. However, they also included a prospective series of 42 children who underwent femoral artery catheterization. In ten of them (24%) the ankle brachial pressure index fell to 0.34 ± 0.33, indicating arterial injury. This is probably a minimal figure, as a rather advanced stenosis must be present before ankle pressure is influenced, at least at rest. In this series ten injuries were seen after umbilical artery catheterization and five after various types of surgical procedures.

Thus, by far the predominating cause of iatrogenic injuries in children is femoral artery catheterization for various indications, other causes being rare. Barr et al. (1977) analyzed infants with less than 1000 g body weight who required peripheral artery catheters, mostly radial, and found no case of clinically apparent peripheral embolism, but there was partial or complete occlusion in more than 80%, as judged by simple palpation or a modified Allen's test. As an alternative route the temporal artery has sometimes been used. Prian (1977) reported on 115 catheterizations where open arteriotomy was used. In six patients there were problems such as retrograde thrombosis of the posterior auricular artery, resulting in severe blanching of the earlobe. Two of these survived with partial loss of the skin along the helix of the earlobe. Prian et al. (1978) also described cerebral embolization after temporal artery catheterization, in one case with permanent hemiparesis. Simmons et al. (1978) raised a warning after they had experienced three cases in which infants developed major hemiplegia contralateral to a temporal artery cutdown. The symptoms did not manifest themselves, however, until the patients were 6 months of age, the catheterization having been performed in the postpartum period.

Fellows (1972) found five patients with persistent but asymptomatic decrease of peripheral pulses after 205 percutaneous transluminal arteriographies in children and one case of reversible peripheral kidney embolization.

Stanger et al. (1974) analyzed the various complications that arose after cardiac catheterization in 1160 patients below the age of 15 years, 218 of them less than 1 month old. By their definitions there were 34 major (three deaths included) and 136 minor complications. Of the major ones, six were arterial thrombosis requiring surgical exploration. In 18 cases there were weak or absent pulses, but as the extremities were warm and with good capillary filling no further treatment was instituted, and the complication was considered minor. The frequency of arterial complications varied considerably with the method of arterial entry. Thus, percutaneous catheterization was associated with fewer complications than was open arteriotomy. Complications were particularly common after brachial arteriotomy, especially in patients with coarctation of the aorta (16.1% vs 3.4%) in patients without coarctation. Jacobsson et al. (1980) also found a considerably higher frequency of thrombosis after angiography through an exposed artery than using a percutaneous approach. Ho et al. (1972) reported 83 arterial thrombi among 1859 cardiac catheterizations (4.5%) in children below the age of 15 years.

One very special cause of injury is catheterization of the umbilical artery in newborn children, and this will be further discussed.

Problems Related to Umbilical Artery Catheterization

Umbilical artery catheterization was introduced by James (1959) and Nelson et al. (1962) as a way to reach the aortoiliac system (Fig. 1). The indications are exchange transfusion, blood pressure measurements, blood sampling, infusion of nutrients and fluids, heart catheterization and angiocardiography. In 1963, in a letter to the Lancet, Ainsworth et al. commented on their experience of 50 catheterizations. Twenty children died, but none from complications of the catheter. In two of them thrombosis around the catheter was found at autopsy. In the same year, in another letter, Cottom (1963) reported no complications whatsoever. In 1966 Anderson et al. described a case of thrombosis around the catheter and intestinal gangrene as a consequence. Cochran et al. (1968) reported on 387 umbilical artery catheterization and noticed vasospasm or blanching of the extremities in 13 cases. In 18 autopsies thrombosis, arteritis, or inflammatory changes were found, and in three cases there was a periarterial hemorrhage. In Larroche's (1970) autopsy series of 77 umbilical artery catheterizations 48% of the patients had thrombosis, and in that of Tyson et al. (1976) thrombosis was found in 33 of 56 autopsies (59%). Egan and Eitzman (1971) performed 259 catheterizations and found 16 clinical and 12 additional autopsy-verified complications (among 68 autopsies) related to the catheter. In five patients there was loss of peripheral

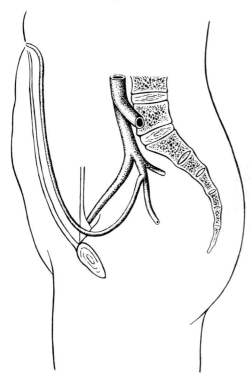

Fig. 1. The arterial system of a new-born with the umbilical artery branching from the internal iliac artery

pulse, in two of them with unilateral gangrene. In six of the autopsy cases there was thrombosis, in two with severe visceral infarction leading to death. Cochran (1976) made an attempt to establish the incidence by sending a questionnaire to 243 hospitals in the United States, but only 94 of the 145 questionnaires returned contained relevant statistics. The data covered 8500 umbilical artery catheterizations, however. Without giving the mortality, he calculated that 30% of children coming to autopsy exhibited thrombotic complications, 6% of which were emboli to the kidneys.

Complications leading to death after umbilical artery catheterization were seen in 0.7% of cases (Johns et al. 1972), but only rarely were these thrombotic complications. Neal et al. (1972; the same analysis was also published by Williams et al. 1972) carried out the first prospective study concerning catheter-induced thrombosis. In a consecutive series of patients, 21 were randomized to undergo pull-out aortography. Eighteen of them had distinct thrombotic alterations, one was normal, and in two cases the technical quality of the investigation was suboptimal. They described four types of clots: pericatheter sheath, irregular pericatheter clot, mural clot, and a combination of pericatheter and mural clot. In most cases the clot embolized at pull-out. Marsh et al. (1975) performed autopsies on 431 infants, 165 of whom had had umbilical artery catheters. In 60% there were pericatheter fibrin sheaths. Arterial thrombosis had caused visceral infarction or limb ischemia in 12 cases. Goetzman et al. (1975) performed aortography in 107 of 215 patients with umbilical artery catheters, nine of the investigations being technically unsatisfactory. In 23 of the 48 satisfactory cases (24%), thrombi were found, fourteen of which only involved the catheter. During the same period there were 32 autopsies and in 21% thromboses were found. In one of the 215 cases the catheter-induced thrombosis was considered the immediate cause of intestinal infarction and perforation. A similar frequency of thrombosis (30%) was found angiographically in a prospective investigation carried out by Olinksy et al. (1975). In their patients there were no clinical signs referable to thrombus formation. Also using angiography, Wesström et al. (1979) found a similar frequency of thrombosis among their 71 patients (26%). Strauss et al. (1974), however, found a much higher angiographic frequency (91%).

Oppenheimer et al. (1982) used ultrasound screening of 71 infants with umbilical artery catheters. Twelve (17%) had clinically evident signs of catheter-induced vascular complications such as blanching, cyanosis, and loss of pulse. In ten of these there were abnormal intraluminal echoes in the aorta and/or common iliac arteries. Among those without clinical signs of ischemia there were two who had fixed intra-aortic abnormalities detected by ultrasound. Interesting in this study was the follow-up with ultrasound in eight children. There was a return to the normal state 2–14 days after catheter removal.

Alpert et al. (1980) analyzed a series of 1461 critically ill infants, 507 of whom had undergone umbilical artery catheterization. In five cases a limb was threatened: two infants died of their main illness but with gangrene, one survivor underwent below-knee amputation, and two infants survived with normal legs after heparinization. O'Neill et al. (1981) reported their experience of approximately 4000 catheterizations. A large number of the patients (the exact figure was not given) had minor ischemic complications prompting removal of the catheter, and 41 had major thromboembolic problems requiring surgical management.

Wharton's jelly embolism from laceration and fragmentation of the arterial wall has been described as a cause of death by Abramowsky et al. (1980). Following this autopsy finding, the authors took kidney samples from 100 consecutive neonatal autopsies and found hemorrhagic and necrotic lesions in 30%, but none with Wharton's jelly. It is not clear from their publication, however, whether or not these neonates all had been catheterized.

A *catheter embolus* to the aorta from a broken umbilical artery catheter has been reported, but this is exceedingly rare (Taber et al. 1973).

Another type of complication may occur because of *catheter perforation*, sometimes with severe hemorrhage as a consequence. There are two sites where perforation is most likely to occur: at the anulus umbilicalis and near the the exit of the umbilical artery from the hypogastric artery (Miller et al. 1979).

The development of *mycotic aneurysm* after umbilical artery catheterization is probably a combined effect of catheter-tip trauma and bacterial infection, usually by *Staphylococcus aureus* (Drucker et al. 1986).

Pathology and Risk Factors

As already mentioned, Aisworth et al. (1963) made the observation of characteristic extensive hemorrhage into the outer part of the arterial wall in newborns with umbilical artery catheters. Chidi et al. (1983) carried out an experimental study in which umbilical artery catheters were inserted into the rabbit aorta for periods of 1 h to 7 days. At various intervals from 1 to 150 days the rabbits were killed and autopsy was performed. There was endothelial disruption in all cases studied within 24 h. Rapid healing was observed when the duration of catheterization was short, but healing was protracted with longer periods of catheterization. Nonocclusive thrombi were frequently found in the aorta. Tyson et al. (1976) did clinicopathologic autopsy studies of 56 children who had had umbilical artery catheters, 33 of them with various stages of thrombosis. The earliest changes within the arteries were platelet fibrin thrombi in areas with abraded vascular endothelium, presumably caused by contact with the catheter. In older infants there was fat within the thrombus, the medial architecture was disrupted, and between the cells there was an excess of acid mucopolysaccharides. Thereafter, varying stages of organization were seen, and in older lesions there were edematous, elevated, fibrous plaques, in one instance with calcium deposits. All such lesions contained stainable fat, mostly as small deposits. Emboli with similar findings as in the aortic lesions were considered to have emanated from the aortic thrombus. There were 113 emboli in the 33 cases; the organs that most frequently were the target for embolism were the intestines, adrenals, liver, lower limbs, pancreas, and kidneys.

There are at least three factors of importance for the development of thrombosis in patients with umbilical artery catheterization. First, an intimal trauma is caused by the catheter. Second, the catheter itself induces platelet aggregation and fibrin deposition. Third, the disease indicating catheterization often induces a thrombogenic state. Goetzman et al. (1975) and Wesström et al. (1979) investigated potential risk factors. Goetzman et al. (1975) found no correlation between duration of catheterization and occurrence of thrombosis. They made a comparison with those cases without thrombosis and found no differences in weight, sex, gestational age, average duration of catheterization, number of catheters, or type of hospital. However, 39% of patients with thrombosis had had leg blanching against 7% of those without. In infants with and without thrombosis Wesström et al. (1979) found no significant differences for gestational age, birth weight, Apgar score, degree of illness, duration of catheterization, or infusion of bicarbonate. These findings were in keeping with data provided by Tyson et al. (1976), who were unable to identify clinical risk factors for the development of thrombi after umbilical artery catheterization.

As already pointed out (p. 168), the patients who need umbilical artery catheters also have a number of risk factors which make the catheterization potentially hazardous. To decrease the risk, several factors can be influenced by the neonatologist:
1. Position of the catheter in the aorta – a factor which is somewhat disputed among neonatologists, however. Mokrohisky et al. (1978) performed a prospective randomized study on the effect of placement of the catheter. A higher complication rate was found in the group with the catheter tip at the third-to-fourth lumbar segment as compared with those with the tip at the seventh-to-eighth thoracic segment. In a similar prospective randomized study of 88 children, Feinauer et al. (1975) found more serious complications in connection with a high position of the catheter, and this was further supported after 213

children had been observed (Feinauer 1979). Wesström et al. (1979) found
fewer thrombi when long catheters were used (Th6–11) than when short ones
were used (L3–5).

2. Type of catheter. In the same study as mentioned above, Wesström et al.
   (1979) found that catheters with an end hole were better than those with side
   holes. Kitterman et al. (1970) found that soft catheters prevented perforation.
3. Catheter material. Boros et al. (1975b) found reduced thrombus formation
   with silicone elastomere compared with polyvinylchloride. Hecker (1981)
   showed marked differences in thrombogenicity between various umbilical artery catheters investigated experimentally in sheep aorta.
4. Indwelling time. Symansky and Fox (1972) and Marsh et al. (1975) found a
   longer duration of catheterization in cases with complications, whereas others
   (Neal et al. 1972; Wesström et al. 1979; Dorand et al. 1977) found no such relation to time.
5. Repeated catheter manipulation (Marsh et al. 1975).
6. Composition of infusate. Hypertonic or otherwise irritating substances (bicarbonate, calcium gluconate, dextrose, amino acids, antibiotics) may damage the
   endothelium (Wigger et al. 1970; Dorand et al. 1977; Mokrohisky et al. 1978;
   Purohit et al. 1978; Seibert et al. 1987; Stringel et al. 1985) and thereby increase
   the tendency for thrombus formation. Direct injection of a hypertonic solution
   into the umbilical artery has led to buttock necrosis (Ortonne et al. 1978), as
   has umbilical artery catheterization (Cutler and Stretcher 1977).
7. Hereditary antithrombin-III deficiency can be treated with administration of
   antithrombin-III concentrate.

As is clear from the above discussion, there is a large variation in the frequency of thrombotic complications, and there is also a discrepancy between
angiographic findings and clinical symptoms of thromboembolism. Moreover,
most data are based on retrospective investigations.

Symptoms and Signs

Symptoms and signs of complications after femoral artery catheterization are discussed in the chapter on angiographic complications (p. 8). What should be remembered is the higher frequency of complications and the greater diagnostic
difficulties in small children. The symptoms are often mild and atypical, which
delays the diagnosis. Birkin and Amplatz (1972) reported on a newborn male infant who sustained a so-called jet collapse of the thoracic aorta during angiography, with disruption of the media and extravasation of the contrast medium and
hematoma formation in the wall. This was ascribed to the injection pressure being too high through an end-hole catheter, causing negative forces in the jet of
the injected contrast medium which may induce collapse of the pliable aortic wall
of newborns. In rare cases of arterial puncture an arteriovenous fistula may develop (Bical et al. 1982).

In cases of umbilical artery catheterization the leg discoloration and blanching
indicate thrombosis (Du et al. 1970; Goetzman et al. 1975). In severely diseased

children, however, blanching can occur although no arterial lesions are found at autopsy (Gupta et al. 1968). Sudden pallor, cold skin, and poor capillary and venous filling should always lead to the suspicion of thrombosis. It is very difficult to discover partial loss of muslce power, pain, anesthesia, and paralysis in infants. Difficulty in maintaining catheter patency is a warning sign that an occlusion is developing. There may also be ischemia in the form of microembolization from a proximally situated thrombus (Alpert et al. 1980; Gupta et al. 1968; Kitterman et al. 1970; Neal et al. 1972; White et al. 1968; Stringel et al. 1985).

Flanigan et al. (1982) reported difficulties in feeding, mottling of the lower half of the body, tachypnea, upper-extremity hypertension, paleness, and no femoral pulses in a 9-day-old child. Acute neonatal congestive heart failure in children with umbilical artery catheterization can be a sign of acute aortic thrombosis (Henry et al. 1981; Flanigan et al. 1982; McFadden and Ochsner 1983; Kreuger et al. 1985; Himmel et al. 1986) or of renal artery thrombosis with renovascular hypertension (Adelman et al. 1978).

In cases of thrombotic occlusion of the celiac or mesenteric arteries intestinal infarction may develop, with perforation and peritonitis (Castleman et al. 1973; Goetzman et al. 1975; O'Neill et al. 1981). Andersson et al. (1974) described a case of cecal perforation probably caused by a peripheral embolus from an umbilical artery catheter thrombus. There is one single report of intestinal perforation due to avulsion of the omphalomesenteric duct remnant upon withdrawal of an umbilical artery catheter (Hoekstra et al. 1977). Thrombotic occlusion of the abdominal aorta and its major visceral branches has been responsible for the development of neonatal necrotizing enterocolitis in some patients, also with a fatal outcome (Joshi et al. 1975; Lehmiller and Kanto 1978; Lividaditis et al. 1974).

Several authors have reported renal artery occlusion at autopsy in children with umbilical artery catheters (Gupta et al. 1968; Johns et al. 1972; Klein et al. 1982; Larroche 1970; Marsh et al. 1975; Wigger et al. 1970). Renovascular hypertension, which develops very early in life, may be a sign of renal artery thrombosis due to umbilical artery catheterization (Adelman et al. 1978; Bergqvist et al. 1987; Brill et al. 1985; Ford et al. 1974).

Merten et al. (1978) described 12 infants with hypertension and held it probable that the just-described mechanism was the cause in five cases. A detailed analyzis of their observations is not possible, however. The children were treated conservatively and at least the short-term result was good. Plumer et al. (1976) suggested umbilical arterial catheterization as the etiologic factor in seven or eight of ten cases of infant hypertension. Five of the children died and three were nephrectomized. O'Neill et al. (1981) mentioned two cases without giving any details. One was relieved of the hypertension after aortic thrombectomy. The other had bilateral renal artery stenoses, one of which was thrombectomized, but hypertension remained. Bauer et al. (1975) reported a case of congestive heart failure. The patient had a palpable left kidney which could not be visualized on excretory urography. An aortography showed an aortic thrombus extruding into the left renal artery and superior mesenteric artery. Heparinization was instituted, but because of sustained hypertension despite intensive medical therapy a nephrectomy was performed, and this normalized the blood pressure. Malloy and Nichols (1977) found a silent left kidney when they investigated a mycotic aneurysm, and hypertension was relieved with a nephrectomy. Aortic thrombi extending into the renal arteries should be removed in cases where surgery is performed, otherwise severe hypertension may be the result (Kreuger et al. 1985). Adelman et al. (1978) reported on a series of 400 critically ill children, 250 of whom underwent umbilical artery catheterization, all without heparinization. Hypertension was diagnosed in nine infants, eight of whom had had umbilical catheters, which corresponded to an incidence of 3.2% in catheterized and 0.7% in noncatheterized infants. The symptoms were rather dramatic, including congestive heart failure in seven. Angiograms were abnormal in six of seven adequately studied, and in the seventh the angiography was not performed until the age of 3 months. All were treated conservatively with large doses of antihypertensive agents. Blood pressure returned to normal in all and remained normal after discontinuation of the medication. The authors concluded that surgery is rarely required.

Bergqvist et al. (1987) reported on a 2-year-old male child with severe hypertension and occlusion of the renal artery, probably as a result of umbilical artery catheterization during the neonatal period. He became symptom free after a nephrectomy.

Aziz and Robertson (1973) reported a case of paraplegia after exchange transfusion. Shortly after the exchange procedure was completed the infant became mottled from 2 cm above the umbilicus and distally, but it had normal pulsations. Twenty-four hours later complete paralysis was diagnosed, and this remained practically unchanged after 1 year. The cause was suggested to be ischemic necrosis of the thoracic spinal cord around the tenth thoracic vertebra on the basis of a catheter-induced thrombosis or embolization. Two further such cases were described by Krishnamoorthy et al. (1976).

Thrombosis or embolism of the inferior gluteal artery, supplying the sciatic nerves as well as the skin of the buttocks, coccygeal area, and upper posterior part of the thigh, may cause foot-drop (Purohit et al. 1978); it may also give rise to the development of necrosis in the gluteal region (Cutler and Stretcher 1977; Purohit et al. 1978; Rudolph et al. 1974).

A few cases of hemoperitoneum after perforation of the aorta or the iliac arteries have been described (Caeton and Goetzman 1985; Johns et al. 1972; Hilliard and Schreiner 1979; Marsh et al. 1975). O'Neill et al. (1981) reported one case in which the common iliac artery was avulsed. Out of 400 umbilical artery catheterizations Miller et al. (1979) reported seven patients with severe extra- and intraperitoneal hemorrhage. The clinical picture always involved hypotension, abdominal distension, and lower abdominal wall ecchymosis. Hematocrit usually declined. Abdominal roentgenograms showed bulging flanks and intraperitoneal fluid. Intra-abdominal hemorrhage has also been observed as a complication of umbilical vein catheterization (Kanto and Parrish 1977). Perforation without bleeding is another possibility (van Leeuwen and Patney 1969), as is intrathoracic perforation (Vidyasagar et al. 1970).

Mycotic aneurysms in the thoracic or abdominal aorta or iliac arteries of 21 patients have been described in some detail; eight patients were female, eleven male, and two were of unreported gender (Spangler et al. 1977; Thompson et al. 1980; Wynn et al. 1982; Stevens and Mandell 1978; Brill et al. 1985; Faer and

Taybi 1977; Fays and Bretagne 1980; Bergsland et al. 1984; Marchal et al. 1978; Malloy and Nichols 1977; Rajs et al. 1976; Rabin et al. 1986; Saabye et al. 1986; Drucker et al. 1986; Wind et al. 1982). The aneurysm was diagnosed at a median time of 4 months after catheterization (1 week–5 years). In all cases there had been infectious complications during catheterization with positive blood cultures. In all cases but one (Drucker et al. 1986) there were various types of staphylococci and in one case *Escherichia coli* and in one *Klebsiella* were found as well. In one case (Drucker et al. 1986) only *Klebsiella* could be grown. Eight cases were detected at autopsy. As a curiosity it can be mentioned that the two cases reported by Marchal et al. (1978) involved female twins; both died, one because of rupture of the mycotic aneurysm. Of the others two were not treated, and the long-term results are unknown. The remaining eleven were operated on: one with resection and end-to-end anastomosis, one with division and ligation of a fistulous communication between the pseudoaneurysm and the common iliac artery, one with lateral closure, and the others with various types of synthetic grafts. All left the hospital alive but the follow-up times are short, and long-term results are not known. O'Neill et al. (1981) reported on another patient with a ruptured mycotic aneurysm who died on the operating table, but no further details are given. In a patient described by Rabin et al. (1986) there were three mycotic aneurysms, and in another multiple aneurysms were found (Bergsland et al. 1984). Typical symptoms have been recurrent cough, bronchitis, pneumonia, and failure to thrive. On chest roentgenograms a mediastinal tumor has been observed, and further investigations have led to the detection of the mycotic aneurysm. Iliac artery aneurysm has always presented as a palpable mass (Drucker et al. 1986). One somewhat special type of aneurysm was reported by Colclough and Barson (1981), in which the aneurysm, detected at autopsy, had a smooth intimal surface, but there was an abrupt loss of the media and elastic tissue at the orifice of the aneurysm. The girl died at 14.5 weeks of age and had had an umbilical artery catheter during her first 26 days of life. Several severe septic complications occurred, *Pseudomonas* being the most persistent pathogen.

Todd et al. (1984) reported on a child with uncomplicated umbilical artery catheterization who at the age of 6 months developed an aneurysm in the left common iliac artery, which was resected. However, microscopic investigation showed the picture of a true aneurysm, indicating that the etiology probably is not the catheter. An umbilical artery pseudoaneurysm was described by Katz et al. (1986), the main symptom of which was a palpable suprabic mass.

Choi et al. (1977) reported two cases of broken umbilical artery catheters. In one case the removed catheter was shorter than expected and the residual part of it was verified on a roentgenogram. It was successfully removed via the common iliac artery. In the other patient the broken catheter was noted on a roentgenogram in the thoracic aorta, but because of the severe respiratory distress syndrome thoracotomy was considered to be contraindicated. The infant died of her primary disease. Successful removal of a broken catheter was described by Lackey and Taber (1972) and Wagner et al. (1987). In the latter case, however, there were embolic complications to the right leg with irreversible sequelae.

Long-Term Sequelae

After Femoral Catheterization

There has been concern about whether or not a femoral artery thrombosis in children may give rise to impaired growth in terms of length. This might be due to decreased blood flow to the muscles of the extremities, which is known from cases of poliomyelitis (Ring 1957) and to a decreased blood supply to the epiphyseal region. Overgrowth of extremities harboring large hemangiomas or arteriovenous fistulas is also known, and this knowledge has been used therapeutically (Hiertonn 1957). It is well known that children operated on with the Blalock-Taussig procedure for Fallot's tetralogy developed a shorter arm on the side of the ligated artery, the length of the radius being diminished and the muscle mass being decreased, whereas subcutaneous fat sometimes increased in thickness (Harris et al. 1964; Currarino and Engle 1964).

Vlad et al. (1964) reinvestigated 500 children who had undergone a total of 542 left heart catheterizations and found only a single patient with postcatheterization peripheral vascular insufficiency. Bassett et al. (1968) investigated 28 children 1–8 years after they had been catheterized at the age of 1 day to 14 years. Twenty-four of the children had diminished leg length as well as a decrease in peripheral pulses and oscillometry. The decrease in length was more than 0.3 cm and involved primarily the tibia. The degree of leg shortening roughly parallelled the severity of circulatory impairment as measured oscillometrically or by diminshed pulses. However, Rosenthal et al. (1972) found no difference in length in 109 heart catheterized patients irrespective of age, type of arterial procedure, or duration of follow-up; 9.6% had diminished pulses but no difference in leg length.

Jacobsson et al. (1973) reexamined 33 children 2–9 years after femoral artery catheterization. Diminished pulses were seen on oscillometry in 12 patients, seven of whom had symptoms in their legs during exercise. Five were reangiographed; four of them were found to have occlusions of the common femoral artery and one a partial obstruction of the superficial femoral artery. Eight underwent plethysmography and had a flow diminishment compared with the noncatheterized leg of 23% (4%–50%). Similar findings have been made using the xenon 133 clearance technique (Skovranek and Samanek 1979), independent of whether Seldinger's percutaneous technique, arteriotomy, or cannulation had been used for cardiac catheterization an average of 2.7 years previously. Bloom et al. (1974) reported on three patients with occlusion of the external iliac artery after heart catheterization. The arteries were reconstructed with bovine carotid heterografts with good immediate results; long-term results are unknown.

Mortensson (1976) reangiographed 44 children, all on strict medical indications, 2 months–9 years after primary angiography. Thirty-seven were normal and seven occluded. All had been younger than 8 years at the primary angiography. Rubenson et al. (1979) found six thromboses among 253 patients who had percutaneous angiography (2.4%). Five underwent a Fogarty procedure and one was heparinized. At follow-up, two had died and four had normal circulation. During the same period Rubenson et al. performed angiography on 14 patients with arterial cutdown and found eight thrombi (57%). Four underwent a Fogarty procedure, two were treated with streptokinase and heparin, and two died before treatment. At follow-up three were normal and three were without clinical symptoms but had decreased oscillometric pulsations. Smith and Green (1981) collected 15 cases from the literature with objectively verified angiographic thrombosis and a follow-up of 0.5–7 years. In 14 of these cases there were growth abnormalities.

After Umbilical Artery Catheterization

Powers and Swyer (1975) performed plethysmographic examinations of 28 children, 29–135 days old, who had all had postbirth umbilical artery catheters and found no difference in flow between the legs. Boros et al. (1975a) reexamined 14 children 4 years after umbilical artery catheterization, and ten of them had a pull-out arteriographic thrombosis but failed to demonstrate any long-term sequelae

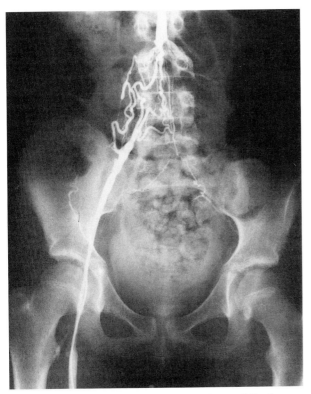

Fig. 2. An 11-year-old female patient had an umbilical artery catheter as a newborn because of prematurity. She then had left leg ischemia, later developing left-sided osteomyelitis and leg shortening. At school age coldness and claudication appeared. As her femoral pulses were very weak, angiography was performed, showing aortic occlusion with a rich collateral network. Reconstruction with a bifurcation graft resulted in an uneventful postoperative course

(pulsations, length, anamnestic data). Wesström (1979) made clinical and plethysmographic examination of 49 children, age 18 (17–28) months, who had had umbilical artery catheters. Angiography during infancy had shown thromboembolism in 14 of them. All the children had higher pressure in the legs than in the arms. Only one child had a pressure difference between the legs of more than 10 mm Hg. One child had a difference in calf circumference of 1.5 cm. That many intravascular alterations are reversible after catheter removal has been demonstrated with ultrasound follow-up by Oppenheimer et al. (1982).

Bergqvist et al. (1987) reported on an 11-year-old girl with several complications from her umbilical artery catheter during the infant period. By and by, she developed rather severe intermittent claudication, and angiography showed an aortic occlusion (Fig. 2). She underwent reconstruction with an aorto-femoral bifurcation graft and the result was good.

Problems concerning renovascular hypertension and mycotic aneurysms have already been discussed above.

Prevention

A primary step in prevention is to take account of the risk factors discussed above. In cases of umbilical artery catheterization, proper catheter placement is important. When a low aortic position is used there may be more complications but they are definitely less severe than when a high position is used (Tooley 1972). When the catheter is placed high there may be visceral necrosis (O'Neill et al. 1981; Vidyasagar et al. 1970). Baker et al. (1969) and Vidyasagar et al. (1970) recommended roentgenographic control to make sure that the tip was placed in the lower aorta. Although there is no complete agreement on the position issue, a control roentgenogram is strongly recommended (Weber et al. 1974). It is probably important that the tip of the catheter not lies adjacent to major arterial branches (Stavis and Krauss 1980). In rare cases the catheters may turn downward in the hypogastric artery with the risk of causing gangrene of the buttock because of thrombosis of the gluteal arteries (Cutler and Stretcher 1977; Purohit et al. 1978; Rudolph et al. 1974). With real-time ultrasound it is also possible to accurately detect the position of the umbilical artery catheter relative to internal vascular structures (Oppenheimer and Carroll 1982).

More complications are seen after long duration of catheterization, but complications have also been reported after a short-term procedure (Alpert et al. 1980). Keen monitoring of blanching, cyanosis, difficulties with aspiration, and diminished pulses must be done. If the catheter is no longer needed or in cases of complications it should be removed immediately.

Special care must be taken with children who are known to have a family history of, e.g., antithrombin-III deficiency, in whom spontaneous neonatal aortic thrombosis may also develop (Bjarke et al. 1974).

When the condition of a critically ill neonate with an umbilical artery catheter deteriorates unexpectedly, aortic thrombosis or hemoperitoneum are two of the differential diagnoses that should be kept in mind.

Silastic catheters should probably be used. This view is based on a nonrandomized study by Boros et al. (1975 b), who performed pull-out aortography in patients with PVC catheters and found 90% with thrombosis, and in patients with silastic (Silicone elastomere) catheters and found only 10% with thrombosis.

In cases of cardiac catheterization through an arterial cutdown it may be beneficial to administer papaverine topically (Izukawa et al. 1968).

Heparinization might be considered (Horgan et al. 1987). Freed et al. (1974) made a randomized study of heparinization in patients undergoing heart catheterization. One hundred and sixty-one patients were randomized, but only in the 77 children who were ten years or younger were thrombotic complications (via oscillometry and clinical examination) seen. The frequency of thrombosis diminished from 40% to 8% when 1 mg/kg body wt. of heparin was given. The frequency of embolectomies decreased from 7/37 in the placebo group to 0/40 in the heparin group. However, Marsh et al. (1975) warned against the use of heparin in neonates, and especially in diseased neonates, because of common intracranial hemorrhage. In cases of umbilical artery catheterization the use of heparin is a matter of controversy. Tooley (1972) and Olinsky et al. (1975) recommended 1 unit/ml in the catheter infusate. Rajani et al. (1979) made a randomized study comparing heparin (1000 IU/ml) and dextrose. Catheter occlusion occurred in four of 32 patients in the heparinized group and in 19 of 30 in the nonheparinized group ($P < 0.01$). Using a life-table analysis it was possible to determine the half-life of catheter function: It was 7 days in the heparinized group and 2 in the nonheparinized group ($P < 0.01$). Blue toes persisting for more than 8 h were equally frequent in the two groups (28% and 27% respectively).

As far as injuries after angiography and cardiac catheterization are concerned, they should become less common, the better the preoperative noninvasive tests become. Thus, Pate et al. (1987) operated on 44 children with congenital heart disease using preoperative 2-D Doppler echocardiography and no catheterization whatsoever.

Treatment

Today it is possible to perform successful aortic thrombectomies even in neonates (Flanigan et al. 1982). It is important to use microsurgical techniques with magnifying lenses or a microscope and microinstruments. Even when acute ischemic symptoms are absent, frequent reports of decreased length growth must be taken into consideration. Of importance for the decision is also the poor surgical risk, the small vessels, and the localization of the thrombosis. Aortic surgery can be successfully performed, femoropopliteal surgery only rarely. In cases of aortic surgery a transverse incision should be used. In smaller vessels patulous anastomosing is recommended (Whitehouse et al. 1976). Interrupted 6.0–9.0 polypropylene or polydioxanone (PDS) sutures should be used (Ray et al. 1981; Flanigan et al. 1983; Himmel et al. 1986). Fine polyethylene tubing can be used to irrigate and also to aspirate clots from small vessels (Cahill et al. 1967). Because of the tendency to spasm and retraction of vessels, vein grafts must often be used. Gentle

Table 2. Results of vascular surgery in children younger than 2 years of age

Author	Age	Etiology	Diagnosis	Procedure	Result	Follow-up time	Comments
Cahill et al. (1967)	3 m	Fem card cath	Thrombosis	Thrombectomy	Rethrombosis	4 m	
	3 m	Fem card cath	Thrombosis	Thrombectomy	Clinically patent	5 m	
	5 m	Fem card cath	Thrombosis	Thrombect+reconstr	Rethrombosis	4 m	
	7 m	Fem card cath	Thrombosis	Thrombectomy	Rethrombosis	5 m	
	13 m	Fem card cath	Thrombosis	Thrombectomy	Residual stenosis	2 m	
	20 m	Fem card cath	Thrombosis	Thrombectomy	Residual stenosis	6 m	
Flanigan et al. (1983)	NB	UAC	Thrombosis	Transabd thrombect	Good	4 m	Urokinase first tried without success
	NB	UAC	Thrombosis	Transabd thrombect		5 m	
	18 m			Fem patch			
	9 m		Thrombosis	Fem thrombectomy	Good		
	2 y		Thrombosis	Fem thrombectomy		?	
Henry et al. (1981)	NB	UAC	Aortic thrombosis	Thrombectomy	Postop death		
	NB	UAC	Aortic thrombosis	Thrombectomy	Repeat thrombectomy, postop death		
Himmel et al. (1986)	NB	UAC	Thrombosis	Thrombectomy	Good	12 m	
Klein et al. (1982)	5 m	Fem angio	Thrombosis	Thrombectomy	Good	?	
	2 m	Fem card cath	Thrombosis	Thrombect+resection and end-to-end anastomosis	Died in surgery	?	
	7 m	Fem card cath	Thrombosis	Thrombectomy??	Rethrombosis	?	
	2 m	Fem card cath	Thrombosis	Thrombect+resection and end-to-end anastomosis	Died in surgery		
	18 m	Fem card cath at 11 m	Iliac thrombosis	Saphenous vein bypass	Postop death	2 y	
	21 m	Fem card cath at 7 m	Iliac thrombosis	Saphenous vein bypass	Leg length equal	2 y	

Author	Age	Cause	Injury	Treatment	Outcome	Follow-up	Comments
Kreuger et al. (1985)	NB	UAC	Aortorenal thrombosis	Thrombectomy	Gangrene, postop death		
	NB	UAC	Aortofemoral thrombosis	Thrombectomy	Good	10 y	
	NB	UAC	Aortorenal thrombosis	Thrombectomy		50 m	Renal thrombendarterectomy at 15 months
	NB	UAC	Aortorenal thrombosis	Thrombectomy		32 m	Decreased left renal function
	NB	UAC	Aortic thrombosis	Thrombectomy		?	Hepatic dysfunction
	NB	UAC	Aortic thrombosis	Thrombectomy		5 m	Lag ischemia
	NB	UAC	Aortic thrombosis	Thrombectomy		3 weeks	Hypertension
McFadden and Ochsner (1983)	NB	UAC	Aortic thrombosis	Thrombectomy	Nonfunctioning left kidney	14 m	
	NB	UAC	Aortic thrombosis	Thrombectomy + femoral embolectomy	BK amputation	8 m	
Meagher et al. (1979)	24 d	Fem art punct	Thrombosis	Thrombectomy	Loss of 3 toes	?	
O'Neill et al. (1981)	NB	UAC	Aortic thrombosis	Thrombectomy	Good	3 m–6 y	One of the patients has weak femoral pulses
	NB	UAC	Aortorenal thrombosis	Thrombect + renal thrombectomy	Hypertension		
	NB	UAC	Aortic thrombosis	Thrombect + femoral thrombectomy	Good		
	NB	UAC	Aortic thrombosis	Thrombectomy	Postop death		
Perry (1983)	<12 m	Mult fem puncture	Thrombosis	Thrombect + patch	Ankle-brachial index	?	Probably failure, the patient had preop gangrene
	<12 m	Attempt to puncture vein	Thrombosis	Thrombectomy	Gangrene, transmetatarsal amputation		Gangrene, transmetatarsal amputation

Table 2 (continued)

Author	Age	Etiology	Diagnosis	Procedure	Result	Follow-up time	Comments
Smith and Green (1981)	7 m	Fem art punct	Thrombosis	Thrombectomy × 2	Thrombosis, postop death		
	4 m	Arteriography	Thrombosis	Thrombectomy × 2	Patent clinically	8 y	
	11 m	Fem card cath	Thrombosis	Thrombectomy × 2	Thrombosis, patent	4 m (death)	
	11 m	Arteriography	Thrombosis	Thrombectomy + patch	Clinically	6 y	
	9 d	UAC	Thrombosis	Thrombectomy	Thrombosis – re-thrombect + bypass after 3 days	Death after 2 days	
White et al. (1968)	3 m	Thigh injection	Thrombosis	Thrombectomy	Amputation of four toes	2 w	
Whitehouse et al. (1976)	1 m	Arterial monit cath	Thrombosis	Thrombectomy	20 mm Hg blood pressure difference between legs	3 y	
	18 m	Arteriography	Thrombosis	Arterioplasty	Good	5 y	

dilation of the vessels can be done with a Fogarty balloon (Richardson et al. 1981), but vein grafts may easily be overdilated and also develop aneurysms (Stanley; discussion in Richardson et al. 1981). For this reason, some surgeons are hesitant to use vein grafts in children. During surgery, heparinization with 100 IU/kg or dextran-40 is used. In cases of mycotic aneurysm resection is the method of choice, and in the few cases there have been, synthetic grafting with PTFE or dacron has been successful (see p. 176).

Conservative therapy as an alternative to surgery has not been systematically investigated. Flanigan et al. (1983) found a high frequency of normalizing ankle brachial pressure index in patients who were treated with heparin. Various doses have been used, but 1 mg/kg/24 h for 4–5 days may be recommended (Alpert et al. 1980; Flanigan et al. 1983; Perry 1983). Rubenson et al. (1979) tried streptokinase in two cases and Flanigan et al. (1982) urokinase, but further attempts with thrombolysis do not appear to have been made. In cases of occlusion of the femoral artery opinions differ on whether to operate or not. Surgery is technically very difficult but, on the other hand, there is a risk of impaired length growth with occlusion. Smith and Green (1981) concluded that "a child with thrombosis of a femoral artery is virtually certain to suffer growth retardation of the affected leg." Therefore, surgery must be seriously considered. However, the prognosis for children younger than 2 years who undergo vascular surgery is rather depressing, and restenosis or reocclusion has been seen in several cases (for a summary of children operated on before the age of 2 years, see Table 2).

Adelman et al. (1978) showed that aggressive medical treatment of children with catheter-induced renovascular hypertension is possible; blood pressure returned to normal in all cases and remained normal after a mean duration of therapy of 4.2 months (0.5–7 months). Such a conservative attitude has also been advocated by Malin et al. (1985).

Whitehouse et al. (1976) and Klein et al. (1982) have operated on small children with length discrepancy and claudication using saphenous vein bypasses with acceptable results (age at operation 7 months–7 years).

References

Abramnowsky CR, Chrenka B, Fanaroff A (1980) Wharton jelly embolism: an unusual complication of umbilical catheterization. J Pediatr 96:739–741

Adelman RD, Merten D, Vogel J, Goetzman BW, Wennberg RP (1978) Nonsurgical management of renovascular hypertension in the neonate. Pediatrics 62:71–76

Ainsworth RW, Gairnder D, Rack JH, Webb M (1963) Umbilical artery for transfusion. Lancet I:445

Alpert J, O'Donnell JA, Parsonnet V, Brief DK, Brener BJ, Goldenkranz RJ (1980) Clinically recognized limb ischemia in the neonate after umbilical artery catheterization. Am J Surg 140:413–418

Anderson JM, Milner RDG, Strich SJ (1966) Pathological changes in the nervous system in severe neonatal hypoglycaemia. Lancet II:372–375

Andersson Å, Hofer PÅ, Holmlund DEW, Wendel HÅ (1974) Colonic perforation secondary to thrombo-embolus from an umbilical artery catheter. Acta Paediat Scand 63:155–156

Aziz EM, Robertson AF (1973) Paraplegia: a complication of umbilical artery catheterization. J Pediatr 82:1051–1052

Baker DH, Berdon WE, James LS (1969) Proper localization of umbilical arterial and venous catheters by lateral roentgenograms. Pediatrics 43:34–39

Barr PA, Sumners J, Wirtschafter D, Porter RC, Cassady G (1977) Percutaneous peripheral arterial cannulation in the neonate. Pediatrics 59:1058–1061

Bassett FH, Lincoln CR, King TD, Canent RV (1968) Inequality in the size of the lower extremity following cardiac catheterization. South Med J 61:1013–1017

Bauer SB, Feldman SM, Gellis SS, Retik AB (1975) Neonatal hypertension. A complication of umbilical-artery catheterization. N Engl J Med 293:1032–1033

Bergqvist D, Bergentz S-E, Hermansson G, Lundberg HO (1987) Late ischaemic sequelae after umbilical artery catheterization. Br J Surg 74:628–629

Bergsland J, Kawaguchi A, Roland JM, Pieroni DR, Subramanian S (1984) Mycotic aortic aneurysms in children. Ann Thorac Surg 37:314–318

Bical O, Laborde F, Lelcompte Y, Leca F, Hazan E, Neveux JY (1982) Fistulas artério-veineuses iatrogénes du nourrisson. Arch Fr Pediatr 39:691–692

Birkin BB, Amplatz K (1972) Jet collapse with aortic rupture – a complication of umbilical catheter angiography. AJR 116:487–489

Bjarke B, Herin P, Blombäck M (1974) Neonatal aortic thrombosis. Acta Paediatr Scand 63:297–301

Bloom JD, Mozersky DJ, Buckley CJ, Hagood CO (1974) Defective limb growth as a complication of catheterization of the femoral artery. Surg Gynecol Obstet 138:524–526

Boijsen E, Lundström N-R (1968) Percutaneous cardiac catheterization and angiocardiography in infants and children. Am J Cardiol 22:572–575

Boros SJ, Nystrom JF, Thompson TR, Reynolds JW, Williams HJ (1975 a) Leg growth following umbilical artery catheter-associated thrombus formation: a 4-year follow-up. J Pediatr 87:973–976

Boros SJ, Thompson TR, Reynolds JW, Jarvis CW, Williams HJ (1975 b) Reduced thrombus formation with silicone elastomere (Silastic) umbilical artery catheters. Pediatrics 56:981–986

Brill PW, Winchester P, Levin AR, Griffith AY, Kazam E, Zirinsky K (1985) Aortic aneurysm secondary to umbilical artery catheterization. Pediatr Radiol 15:199–201

Caeton J, Goetzman B (1985) Risky business. Umbilical arterial catheterization. Am J Dis Child 139:120–121

Cahill JL, Talbert JL, Ottesen OE, Rowe RD, Haller JA (1967) Arterial complications following cardiac catheterization in infants and children. J Pediatr Surg 2:134–143

Castleman B, Scully RE, McNeely BU (1973) Case records of the Massachusetts general hospital. Case 45-1973. N Engl J Med 289:1027–1033

Chidi CC, King DR, Boles ET (1983) An ultrastructural study of the intimal injury induced by an indwelling umbilical artery catheter. J Pediatr Surg 18:109–115

Choi SJ, Raziuddin K, Haller JO (1977) Broken umbilical artery catheter: a report of two cases. Am J Dis Child 131:595

Cochran WD (1976) Umbilical artery catheterization. 69th Ross Conference on Pediatric Research, Columbus Ohio, pp 28–32

Cochran WD, Davis HT, Smith CA (1968) Advantages and complications of umbilical artery catheterization in the newborn. Pediatrics 42:769–777

Colclough AB, Barson AJ (1981) Infantile aortic aneurysm complicating umbilical arterial catheterisation. Arch Dis Child 56:795–797

Cottom D (1963) Umbilical artery for transfusion. Lancet I:329

Currarino G, Engle MA (1965) The effects of ligation of the subclavian artery on the bones and soft tissues of the arms. J Pediatr 67:808–811

Cutler VE, Stretcher GS (1977) Cutaneous complications of central umbilical artery catheterization. Arch Dermatol 113:61–63

Dorand RD, Cook LN, Andrews BF (1977) Umbilical vessel catheterization. The low incidence of complications in a series of 200 newborn infants. Clin Pediatr 16:569–572

Drucker DEM, Greenfield LJ, Ehrlich F, Salzberg AM (1986) Aorto-iliac aneurysms following umbilical artery catheterization. J Pediatr Surg 21:725–730

Du JNH, Briggs JN, Young G (1970) Disseminated intravascular coagulopathy in hyaline membrane disease: massive thrombosis following umbilical artery catheterization. Pediatrics 45:287–289

Egan EA, Eitzman DV (1971) Umbilical vessel catheterization. Am J Dis Child 121:213–218

Faer MJ, Taybi H (1977) Mycotic aortic aneurysm in premature infants. Pediatr Radiol 125:177–180

Fays J, Bretagne MC (1980) Unusual evolution of a mycotic hypogastric arterial aneurysm after arterial umbilical catheterization. Pediatrics 9:50–52

Feinauer LR (1979) Letter to the editor. N Engl J Med 300:317

Feinauer LR, Atherton SO, Jung AL (1975) High vs low placement of umbilical artery catheters (Abstract). Clin Res 23:158A

Fellows K (1972) The uses and abuses of abdominal and peripheral arteriography in children. Radiol Clin North Am 10:349–366

Flanigan DP, Schuler JJ (1986) Pediatric vascular emergencies. In: Bergan JJ, Yao JST (eds) Vascular surgical emergencies. Grune and Stratton, New York, pp 233–244

Flanigan DP, Stolar CJ, Pringle KC, Schuler JJ, Fisher E, Vidyasager D (1982) Aortic thrombosis after umbilical artery catheterization. Successful surgical management. Arch Surg 117:371–374

Flanigan DP, Keifer TJ, Schuler JJ, Ryan TJ, Castronuovo JJ (1982) Experience with iatrogenic pediatric vascular injuries. Incidence, etiology, management, and results. Ann Surg 198:430–442

Ford KT, Teplick SK, Clark RE (1974) Renal artery embolism causing neonatal hypertension. Pediatr Radiol 113:169–170

Freed MD, Keane JF, Rosenthal A (1974) The use of heparinization to prevent arterial thrombosis after percutaneous cardiac catheterization in children. Circulation 50:565–569

Goetzman BW, Stadalnik RC, Bogren HG, Blankenship W, Ikeda RM, Thayer J (1975) Thrombotic complications of umbilical artery catheters: a clinical and radiographic study. Pediatrics 56:374–379

Goldblom RB, Hillman DA, Santulli T (1967) Arterial thrombosis following femoral venipuncture in edematous nephrotic children. Pediatrics 40:450–451

Gupta JM, Roberton NRC, Wigglesworth JS (1968) Umbilical artery catheterization in the newborn. Arch Dis Child 43:382–387

Harris AM, Segel N, Bishop JM (1964) Blalock-Taussig anastomosis for tetralogy of Fallot. A ten-to-fifteen-year follow-up. Br Heart J 26:266–273

Hecker JF (1981) Thrombogenicity of tips of umbilical catheters. Pediatrics 67:467–471

Henriksson P, Wesström G, Hedner U (1979) Umbilical artery catheterization in newborns. III. Thrombosis – a study of some predisposing factors. Acta Pediatr Scand 68:719–723

Henry CG, Gutierrez F, Lee JT et al. (1981) Aortic thrombosis presenting as congestive heart failure: an umbilical artery catheter complication. J Pediatr 98:829–832

Hiertonn T (1957) Arteriovenous anastomoses and acceleration of bone growth. Acta Orthop Scand 26:322

Hilliard J, Schreiner RL (1979) Hemoperitoneum associated with exchange transfusion through an umbilical arterial catheter. Am J Dis Child 133:216

Himmel PD, Sumner DS, Mongkolsmai C, Khanna N (1986) Neonatal thoracoabdominal aortic thrombosis associated with the umbilical artery catheter: successful management by transaortic thrombectomy. J Vasc Surg 4:119–123

Ho CS, Krovetz LJ, Rowe RD (1972) Major complications of cardiac catheterization and angiocardiography in infants and children. Johns Hopkins Med J 131:247–258

Hoekstra RE, Semba T, Fangman JJ, Strobel JL (1977) Intestinal perforation following withdrawal of umbilical artery catheter. J Pediatr 90:290

Hohn AR, Craenen J, Lambert EC (1969) Arterial pulses following percutaneous catheterization in children. Pediatrics 43:617–620

Horgan M, Bartoletti A, Polansky S, Peters J, Manning T, Lamont B (1987) Effect of heparin infusates in umbilical arterial catheters on frequency of thrombotic complications. J Pediatr 111:774–778

Izukawa T, Varghese PJ, Rowe RD (1968) Topical papaverine in arteriotomies in infants and children: effect on incidence of thrombosis. J Pediatr 72:853–854

Jacobsson B, Carlgren LE, Hedvall G, Sivertsson R (1973) A review of children after arterial catheterization of the leg. Pediatr Radiol 1:96–99

Jacobsson B, Curtin H, Rubenson A, Sörensen S-E (1980) Complications of angiography in children and means of prevention. Acta Radiol Diagn 21:257–261

James LS (1959) Biochemical aspects of asphyxia at birth. In: Adaptation to extrauterine life. Report of the thirty-first Ross Conference on Pediatric Research, Vancouver, B.C, 1959

Johns AW, Kitchen WH, Leslie DW (1972) Complications of umbilical vessel catheters. Med J Aust 2:810–815

Joshi VV, Draper DA, Bates III RD (1975) Neonatal necrotizing enterocolitis. Arch Pathol 99:540–543

Kanto WP, Parrish RA (1977) Perforation of the peritoneum and intra-abdominal hemorrhage. A complication of umbilical vein catheterizations. Am J Dis Child 131:1102–1103

Katz M, Perlman J, Tack E, McAlister W (1986) Neonatal umbilical artery pseudoaneurysm: sonographic evaluation (case report). AJR 147:322–324

Kitterman JA, Phibbs RH, Tooley WH (1970) Catheterization of umbilical vessels in newborn infants. Pediatr Clin North Am 17:895–912

Klein MD, Coran AG, Whitehouse WM, Stanley JC, Wesley JR, Lebowitz EA (1982) Management of iatrogenic arterial injuries in infants and children. J Pediatr Surg 17:933–939

Kreuger TC, Neblett WW, O'Neill JA, MacDonell RC, Dean RH, Thieme GA (1985) Management of aortic thrombosis secondary to umbilical artery catheters in neonates. J Pediatr Surg 20:328–332

Krishnamoorthy KS, Fernandez RJ, Todres ID, De Long GR (1976) Paraplegia associated with umbilical artery catheterization in the newborn. Pediatrics 58:443–445

Lackey DA, Taber P (1972) An unusual complication of umbilical artery catheterization. Pediatrics 49:281–282

Larroche JC (1970) Umbilical catheterization: its complications. Biol Neonate 16:101–116

Leblanc J, Wood AE, O'Shea M, Williams WG, Trusler GA, Rowe RD (1985) Peripheral arterial trauma in children. A fifteen-year review. J Cardiovasc Surg (Torino) 26:325–331

Lehmiller DJ, Kanto WP (1978) Relationships of mesenteric thromboembolism, oral feeding, and necrotizing enterocolitis. J Pediatr 92:96–100

Livaditis A, Wallgren G, Faxelius G (1974) Necrotizing enterocolitis after catheterization of the umbilical vessels. Acta Paediatr Scand 63:277–282

Malin S, Baumgart S, Rosenberg H, Foreman J (1985) Nonsurgical management of obstructive aortic thrombosis complicated by renovascular hypertension in the neonate. J Pediatr 106:630–634

Malloy MH, Nichols MM (1977) False abdominal aortic aneurysm: an unusual complication of umbilical arterial catheterization for exchange transfusion. J Pediatr 90:285–286

Mansfield PB, Gazzhangia AB, Litwin SB (1970) Management of arterial injuries related to cardiac catheterization in children and young adults. Circulation 42:501–507

Marchal C, Couronne M, Rouquier F, Lapierre H, Greff M, Mulot O (1978) Anevrisme aortique, septicemie a staphylocoque et catheterisme arterial ombilical. Arch Fr Pediatr 35:74–81

Marsh JL, King W, Barrett C, Fonkalsrud EW (1975) Serious complications after umbilical artery catheterization for neonatal monitoring. Arch Surg 110:1203–1208

McFadden PM, Ochsner JL (1983) Neonatal aortic thrombosis: complication of umbilical artery cannulation. J Cardiovasc Surg (Torino) 24:1–4

Meagher DP, Defore WW, Mattox KL, Harberg FJ (1979) Vascular trauma in infants and children. J Trauma 19:532–536

Merten DF, Vogel JM, Adelman RD, Goetzman BW, Bogren HG (1978) Renovascular hypertension as a complication of umbilical arterial catheterization. Pediatr Radiol 126:751–757

Miller D, Kirkpatrick BV, Kodroff M, Ehrlich FE, Salzberg AM (1979) Pelvic exsanguination following umbilical artery catheterization in neonates. J Pediatr Surg 14:264–269

Mokrohisky ST, Levine RL, Blumhagen JD, Wesenberg RL, Simmons MA (1978) Low positioning of umbilical-artery catheters increases associated complications in newborn infants. N Engl J Med 299:561–564

Mortensson W (1976) Angiography of the femoral artery following percutaneous catheterization in infants and children. Acta Radiol [Diagn] (Stockh) 17:581–593

Mortensson W, Hallböök T, Lundström N-R (1975a) Percutaneous catheterization of the femoral vessels in children. I. Influence on arterial peak flow and venous emptying rate in the calves. Pediatr Radiol 3:195–200

Mortensson W, Hallböök T, Lundström N-R (1975b) Percutaneous catheterization of the femoral vessels in children. II. Thrombotic occlusion of the catheterized artery: frequency and causes. Pediatr Radiol 4:1–9

Neal WA, Reynolds JW, Jarvis CW, Williams HJ (1972) Umbilical artery catheterization: demonstration of arterial thrombosis by aortography. Pediatrics 50:6–13

Nelson NM, Prod'hom LS, Cherry RB, Lipsitz PJ, Smith CA (1962) Pulmonary function in the newborn infant. II. Perfusion-estimation by analysis of the arterial-alveolar carbon dioxide difference. Pediatrics 30:975–989

Olinsky A, Aitken FG, Isdale JM (1975) Thrombus formation after umbilical arterial catheterization. S Afr Med J 49:1467–1470

O'Neill JA (1983) Traumatic vascular lesions in infants and children. In: Dean RH, O'Neill JA (eds) Vascular disorders of childhood. Lea and Febiger, Philadelphia, pp 181–193

O'Neill JA, Neblett WW, Born ML (1981) Management of major thromboembolic complications of umbilical artery catheters. J Pediatr Surg 16:972–977

Oppenheimer DA, Carroll BA (1982) Ultrasonic localization of neonatal umbilical catheters. Radiology 147:781–782

Oppenheimer DA, Carroll BA, Garth K (1982) Ultrasonic detection of complications following umbilical arterial catheterization in the neonate. Radiology 145:667–672

Ortonne J-P, Jeune R, Souteyrand P, Thivolet J (1978) Cutaneous and urinary complications of central umbilical artery injection. Arch Dermatol 114:286–287

Pate JW, Watson DC, Di Sessa TG (1987) Preoperative noninvasive anatomic and physiologic evaluation in congenital heart disease in children. 32nd World congress of surgery, Sydney, 1987

Perry MO (1983) Iatrogenic injuries of arteries in infants. Surg Gynecol Obstet 157:415–418

Plumer LB, Kaplan GW, Mendoza SA (1976) Hypertension in infants – a complication of umbilical arterial catheterization. J Pediatr 89:802–805

Polesky RE, Harvey JP (1968) Gangrene of the extremity following femoral venipuncture: a report of two cases. Pediatrics 42:676–677

Powers WF, Swyer PR (1975) Limb blood flow following umbilical arterial catheterization. Pediatrics 55:248–256

Prian GW (1977) Complications and sequelae of temporal artery catheterization in the high-risk newborn. J Pediatr Surg 12:829–835

Prian GW, Wright GB, Rumack CM, O'Meara OP (1978) Apparent cerebral embolization after temporal artery catheterization. J Pediatr 93:115–118

Purohit DM, Levkoff AH, deVito PC (1978) Gluteal necrosis with foot-drop. Am J Dis Child 132:897–899

Rabin E, Vye MV, Farrell EE (1986) Umbilical artery catheterization complicated by multiple mycotic aortic aneurysm. Arch Pathol Lab Med 110:442–444

Rajani K, Goetzman BW, Wennberg RP, Turner E, Abildgaard C (1979) Effect of heparinization of fluids infused through an umbilical artery catheter on catheter patency and frequency of complications. Pediatrics 63:552–556

Rajs J, Finnström O, Wesström G (1976) Aortic aneurysm developing after umbilical artery catheterization. Acta Paediatr Scand 65:495–498

Ray JA, Doddi N, Regula D, Williams JA, Melveger A (1981) Polydioxanone (PDS), a novel monofilament synthetic absorbable suture. Surg Gynecol Obstet 153:497–507

Richardson JD, Fallat M, Nagaraj HS, Groff DB, Flint LM (1981) Arterial injuries in children. Arch Surg 116:685–690

Ring PA (1957) Shortening and paralysis in poliomyelitis. Lancet 2:980–983

Rosenthal A, Anderson M, Thomson SJ, Pappas AM, Fyler DC (1972) Superficial femoral artery catheterization. Am J Dis Child 124:240–242

Rubenson B, Jacobsson B, Sorensen S-E (1979) Treatment and sequelae of angiographic complications in children. J Pediatr Surg 14:154–157

Rudolph N, Wang H-H, Dragutsky D (1974) Gangrene of the buttock: a complication of umbilical artery catheterization. Pediatrics 53:106–109

Saabye J, Elbirk A, Smith C (1986) Mycotic aneurysm of the thoracic aorta as a late complication of umbilical artery catheterization. Scand J Thorac Cardiovasc Surg 20:179–182

Seibert J, Taylor B, Williamson S, Szabo J, Corbitt S (1987) Sonographic detection of neonatal umbilical-artery thrombosis: clinical correlation. AJR 148:965–968

Shaker IJ, White JJ, Signer RD, Golladay ES, Haller JA (1976) Special problems of vascular injuries in children. J Trauma 16:863–867

Simmons MA, Levine RL, Lubchenco LO, Guggenheim MA (1978) Clinical note. Warning: serious sequelae of temporal artery catheterization. J Pediatr 92:284

Skovranek J, Samanek M (1979) Chronic impairment of leg muscle blood flow following cardiac catheterization in childhood. AJR 132:71–75

Smith C, Green RM (1981) Pediatric vascular injuries. Surgery 90:20–31

Spangler JG, Kleinberg F, Fulton RE, Barnhorst DA, Ritter DG (1977) False aneurysm of the descending aorta. Am J Dis Child 131:1258–1259

Stanger P, Heymann MA, Tarnoff H, Hoffman JI, Rudolph AM (1974) Complications of cardiac catheterization of neonates, infants, and children. A three-year study. Circulation 50:595–608

Stavis RL, Krauss AN (1980) Complications of neonatal intensive care. Clin Perinatol 7:107–124

Stevens PS, Mandell J (1978) Urologic complications of neonatal umbilical arterial catheterization. J Urol 120:605–606

Strauss AW, Escobedo M, Goldring D (1974) Continuous monitoring of arterial oxygen tension in the newborn infant. J Pediatr 85:254–261

Stringel G, Mercer S, Richler M, McMurray B (1985) Catheterization of the umbilical artery in neonates: surgical implications. Can J Surg 28:143–146

Symansky MR, Fox A (1972) Umbilical vessel catheterization: indications, management, and evaluation of the technique. J Pediatr 5:820–826

Taber P, Lackey D, Mikity V (1973) Roentgenographic findings of complications with neonatal umbilical vascular catheterizations. AJR 118:49–57

Thompson TR, Tilleli J, Johnson DE et al. (1980) Umbilical artery catheterization complicated by mycotic aortic aneurysm in neonates. Adv Pediatr 7:275–318

Todd D, Leigh J, Miller R, Votava H (1984) True aneurysm formation in a 6-month-old child. J Pediatr Surg 19:310–311

Tooley WH (1972) What is the risk of an umbilical artery catheter? Pediatrics 50:1–2

Tyson JE, DeSa DJ, Moore S (1976) Thromboatheromatous complications of umbilical arterial catheterization in the newborn period. Arch Dis Child 51:744–754

Van Leeuwen G, Patney M (1969) Complications of umbilical vessel catheterization: peritoneal perforation. Pediatrics 44:1028–1030

Vidyasagar D, Downes JJ, Boogs TR (1970) Respiratory distress syndrome of newborn infants. Clin Pediatr 9:332–337

Vlad P, Hohn A, Lambert EC (1964) Retrograde arterial catheterization of the left heart. Circulation 29:787–793

Wagner C, Vincour C, Weintraub W (1987) Retrieval of an umbilical artey catheter: a potential for misadventure. South Med J 80:1434–1435

Weber AL, DeLuca S, Shannon DC (1974) Normal and abnormal position of the umbilical artery and venous catheter on the roentgenogram and review of complications. AJR 120:361–366

Wesström G (1979) Umbilical artery catheterization in newborns. Linköping University Medical Dissertations No 81, Linköping University, Sweden

Wesström G, Finnström O, Stenport G (1979) Umbilical artery catheterization in new-borns. I. Thrombosis in relation to catheter type and position. Acta Pediatr Scand 68:575–581

White JJ, Talbert JL, Haller JA (1968) Peripheral arterial injuries in infants and children. Ann Surg 167:757–766

Whitehouse WM, Coran AG, Stanley JC, Kuhns LR, Weintraub WH, Fry WJ (1976) Pediatric vascular trauma. Manifestations, management, and sequelae of extremity arterial injury in patients undergoing surgical treatment. Arch Surg 111:1269–1275

Wigger HJ, Bransilver BR, Blanc WA (1970) Thromboses due to catheterization in infants and children. J Pediatr 76:1–11

Williams HJ, Jarvis CW, Neal WA, Reynolds JW (1972) Vascular thromboembolism complicating umbilical artery catheterization. AJR 116:475–486

Wind ES, Wisoff BG, Baron MG, Balsam D, Gootman N, Harrison D (1982) Mycotic aneurysm in infancy: a complication of umbilical artery catheterization. J Pediatr Surg 17:324–325

Wynn M, Rowen M, Rucker RW, Sperling DR, Gazzaniga AB (1982) Pseudoaneurysm of the thoracic aorta: a late complication of umbilical artery catheterization. Ann Thorac Surg 34:186–191

Subject Index

World Journal of Surgery

Official Journal of the Société Internatio-
nale de Chirurgie, of the Collegium Inter-
nationale Chirurgiae Digestivae, and of
the International Association of Endo-
crine Surgeons

ISSN 0364-2313   Title No. 268

Editor-in-Chief: S. A. Wells, Jr., St. Louis,
MO

World Journal of Surgery provides the
reader with in-depth coverage of recent
surgical developments. Each issue
contains a Progress Symposium – a
feature focusing on a single topic of
current interest to surgeons. Organized by
well-known guest editors, these reports
present invited contributions from recognized authorities and provides the latest
information on major clinical problems in
the field.

Each issue also publishes original reports
on clinical findings from surgeons around
the world, with invited commentary from
a second source: firsthand accounts of the
development of important surgical knowledge and techniques; book reviews,
abstracts, commentaries by members of
the editorial board, and letters to the
editor.

Springer-Verlag Berlin
Heidelberg New York London
Paris Tokyo Hong Kong

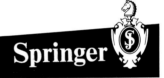

Springer

Surgical and Radiologic Anatomy

ISSN 0930-312X/   Title Nos. 276/286
0930-3138 (with French translations)

Editor-in-Chief: J. P. Chevrel, Paris

Managing Editors: P. Lasjaunias, Paris;
R. Louis, Marseille; R. E. Coupland, Notting-
ham; M. W. Donner, Baltimore

Anatomy is a fundamental science of para-
mount importance in clinical medicine. In
both training and research, the study of
anatomy must therefore be well adapted to
current medical practice.
Surgical and Radiologic Anatomy is designed
to provide clinicians, whether general practi-
tioners, or specialists, surgeons or radiologists,
with information to keep them up to date in
this field and to open up a pathway to the best
possible applications in their particular
specialty.
To meet this goal, each issue contains articles
on the anatomical basis of medical, radiological and surgical techniques, papers on original
research, commentary, and book reviews.
Particular attention is paid to the illustrations
which must be of a high quality so as to be a
real contribution to a better understanding of
anatomical problems. Editions with complete
French translations available.

Springer-Verlag Berlin
Heidelberg New York London
Paris Tokyo Hong Kong

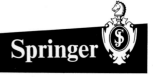

Springer